LOW BACK PAIN SYNDROME

LOW BACK PAIN
SYNDROME
Edition 3

RENE CAILLIET, M.D.

Professor and Chairman
Department of Rehabilitative Medicine
University of Southern California
School of Medicine
Los Angeles, California
Illustrations by R. Cailliet, M.D.

 F. A. DAVIS COMPANY • Philadelphia

Also by Rene Cailliet:

FOOT AND ANKLE PAIN
HAND PAIN AND IMPAIRMENT
KNEE PAIN AND DISABILITY
NECK AND ARM PAIN
SCOLIOSIS
SHOULDER PAIN
SOFT TISSUE PAIN AND DISABILITY

**Library of Congress Cataloging in
Publication Data**

Cailliet, René.
    Low back pain syndrome.

    Includes bibliographies and index.
    1. Backache.   I. Title.
RD768.C3 1981   617'.56   80-15815
ISBN 0-8036-1605-8

Preface

Low back pain remains an enigma of modern society and a great dilemma for the medical profession. Thousands of articles on the subject appear annually in medical journals throughout the world, and numerous theories, techniques, and modalities have been advocated.

The low back pain syndrome affects probably 80 percent of all persons during their lifetime. In most cases the condition spontaneously remits with no residual disability or impairment. Estimates are that 70 percent of patients recover within 1 month, and 90 percent within 3 months, with only 4 percent remaining afflicted for longer than 6 months. Of patients disabled by chronic pain for more than 6 months, only 50 percent return to work.

Numerous developments have occurred since the first edition of this book appeared. The author's experience has served to modify a number of previously held ideas, and many concepts have gained acceptance, tending in the direction of more definitive evaluation and management of low back pain disorders. This third edition is presented in the hope of clarifying these recent advancements.

There can be no change in the concept that precise knowledge of functional anatomy is mandatory in understanding any form of musculoskeletal pain. New ideas emerge, however, to address such questions as how improper function impairs anatomical function, how pain results from these deviations, how pain is transmitted and interpreted, and how various modalities and treatment methods can restore proper function and decrease painful behavior and resultant disability.

An enigma remains in that there is no universality or standardization of low back pain disorders. The term "syndrome" must remain in today's terminology without clarification or universal understanding. Thus low back pain remains a symptom of vague etiology. Numerous terms prevail in the literature along with nonspecific mechanisms and, therefore, nonspecific treatment regimes. Terms such as lumbosacral strain, unstable back, lumbar discogenic disease, facet syndrome, pyriformis syndrome, iliolumbar ligamentous strain, quadratus lumbar pain, myofascitis, spinal stenosis, degenerative disc disease, latissimus dorsi syndrome, abnormal transforaminal ligaments, multifidus triangle syndrome, and a great many more enjoy current vogue.

Each diagnosis is evaluated and treated with varying success. Treatment can include epidural steroid injection, manipulation, rhizotomy, electrocautery, chemical therapy, and facet joint injection, in addition to the time-honored standards of rest, posture training, traction, medication, and systematic exercise.

New terms evolve with time, and new treatments have their advocates, but there is no standardization. Thus the efficacy of any treatment and subjective end results cannot have meaningful statistical value.

Low back pain considered to have existed less than 2 months can be termed acute. The history can identify causation in most instances, and the tissue site of pain can be determined and the treatment reasonably well established. As most acute episodes are self-limited, even arbitrary treatment, or none at all, can be credited.

Chronic back pain, like any chronic pain, may persist in the absence of any clinical findings or confirmatory tests, and in spite of numerous specific treatments. The evaluation and classification of these chronic pain behaviors are the major concern and interest in today's practice. Determination of the patient who will progress into chronic pain behavior, in spite of understood acute pain and in defiance of proper treatment, remains an unsolved need.

Treatment of the acute or the prolonged reaction to acute insult to the low back has a basis in the understood mechanisms and the appreciated personality of the injured person. Adequate evaluation and treatment of acute or subacute and many chronic low back pain syndromes will often diminish the likelihood of full progression into the area of chronic pain. Understanding and recognition of the chronic pain-prone patient will minimize the frequency of this condition with all its attendant socioeconomic sequelae.

This new edition will evaluate current etiologies and mechanisms of acute pain and persistent subacute chronic pain. Treatment modalities will be discussed. The chronic pain problem will be introduced, but more definitive evaluation and treatment of the chronic pain patient will be left to other disciplines. Hopefully this contribution will assist in determining more meaningful terminology, more precise diagnosis, and more specific management.

RENE CAILLIET, M.D.

Contents

Illustrations

CHAPTER 1

Anatomy

The vertebral column is an aggregate of articulated, superimposed segments, each of which is a *functional unit*. The function of the vertebral column is to support a two-legged animal, man, in an upright position, mechanically balanced to conform to the stress of gravity, permitting locomotion and assisting in purposeful movements.

The functional unit is structurally and functionally capable of permitting all these functions through the decades of man's existence. Natural attritional changes of aging, recovery from repeated minor trauma and stresses, impairment from disease or major trauma, and dysfunction from misuse and abuse—all may lead to disability and pain. Its resiliency is a tribute to its structural perfection.

The functional unit is composed of two segments: the anterior segment containing two adjacent vertebral bodies, one superincumbent upon the other, separated by an intervertebral disc, and a posterior neural segment. The anterior segment is essentially a supporting, weight-bearing, shock-absorbing, flexible structure. The posterior segment is a non-weight-bearing structure that contains and protects the neural structures of the central nervous system as well as paired joints that function to direct the movement of the unit (Fig. 1).

ANTERIOR PORTION OF FUNCTIONAL UNIT

The anterior portion of the functional unit is well constructed for its weight-bearing, shock-absorbing function. The unit is comprised of two cylindrical vertebral bodies with flattened cephalic and caudal ends that, in their normal state, are adequate to sustain extremes of compressive stresses. These two vertebral bodies are separated by a hydraulic system called a disc.

At birth the vertebral bodies are bi-convex with the end plates being cartilaginous. These cartilage plates gradually undergo ossification and

1

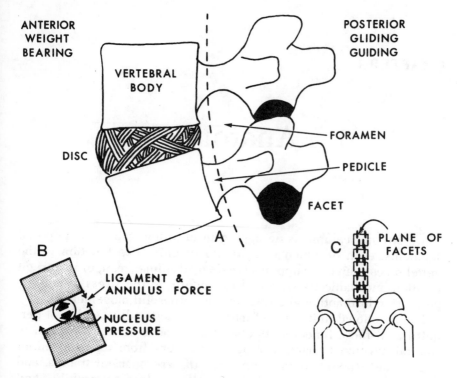

ANTERIOR
WEIGHT
BEARING

VERTEBRAL
BODY

POSTERIOR
GLIDING
GUIDING

DISC

FORAMEN

PEDICLE

FACET

A

B

LIGAMENT &
ANNULUS FORCE

NUCLEUS
PRESSURE

C

PLANE OF
FACETS

FIGURE 1. The functional unit of the spine in cross section. A. Lateral view. B depicts pressures within disc forcing vertebra apart and the balancing force of the long ligaments. C depicts the plane of the facets gliding motion.

from the age of 16 to 20 years fuse with the bony vertebra. This end plate is the point of attachment of the fibers of the annulus fibrosus, and after puberty when ossification is completed, the central and posterior aspects of the plate remain cartilaginous.

The disc is a self-contained fluid system that absorbs shock, permits transient compression, and, owing to fluid displacement within an elastic container, allows movement. It is quite evident then that the disc is a mechanical "shock absorber."

The anatomy of the disc lends itself well to its intended function. The upper and the lower plates of the disc are the end plates of the vertebral bodies. These plates are articular hyaline cartilage in direct contact and adherent to the underlying resilient bone of the vertebral body. In their normal state these end plates are firm, flat, circular, inflexible surfaces that form the cephalad and caudal portions of the disc and to which is attached the encircling annulus fibrosus.

The annulus, or wall, of the disc is an intertwining fibroelastic mesh that encapsulates the matrix of the disc. The matrix, or nucleus pul-

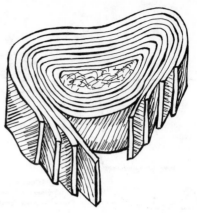

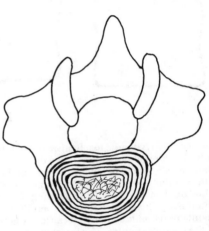

FIGURE 2. Annulus fibrosus. *Above:* Layer concept of annulus fibrosus. *Below:* Circumferential annular fibers about the centrally located pulpy nucleus (nucleus pulposus).

posus, is thus confined within a fibrous resilient wall, the annulus, and between a floor and ceiling composed of the end plates of the vertebrae (Fig. 2). The annulus fibrils are attached around the entire circumference of both the upper and inferior vertebral bodies and crisscross and intertwine in oblique directions. The manner in which these semi-elastic fibers intertwine permits movement of one vertebra upon the other in a rocker-like movement and to a lesser degree permits movement in a shearing direction.

The fluid contained within the confines of the encircling annulus is a colloidal gel and by its self-contained fluidity has all the characteristics of a hydraulic system. Because the nucleus is approximately 88 percent fluid, it cannot itself be compressed, but since it exists in a closed container, it conforms to the law of Pascal (Blaise Pascal, 1623-1662), which states that: "Any external force exerted on a unit area of a confined liquid is transmitted undiminished to every unit area of the interior of the containing vessel."

The self-contained fluid accepts the shock of a compression force

3

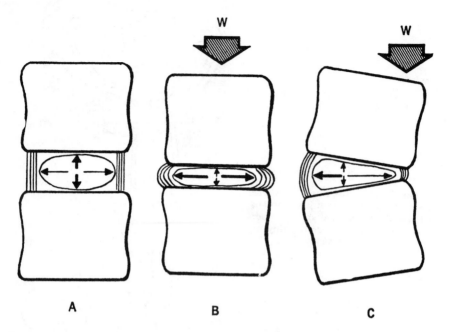

FIGURE 3. Hydraulic mechanism of the intervertebral disc. A. The normal resting disc with the internal pressure indicated by the arrows exerted in all directions. The disc is confined above and below by the vertebral plates and circumferentially by the annulus. The annulus fibers are taut. B. Compression of the disc is permitted by the noncompressible fluid of the nucleus expanding the annulus. Flexibility is seen to exist in the annulus. C. Flexion of the spine is permitted by horizontal shift of the nuclear fluid which maintains its cubic content but causes expansion of the posterior annulus and contraction of the anterior annulus. The intertwining of the annular fibers permits this change in the capsule with no loss of turgor.

attempting to approximate the two vertebrae and maintains the separation of the two vertebral bodies. Movement of one vertebra on the other in a rocking-like manner is permitted by the ability of the fluid to shift anteriorly or posteriorly within a semielastic container (Fig. 3). The constant internal disc pressure separates the two end plates and thus keeps the fibroelastic mesh of the annulus taut (Fig. 4).

The elastic properties of the disc are considered to reside in the elasticity of the annulus rather than in the fluid content of the nucleus. In a "young" and undamaged disc the fibroelastic tissue of the annulus is predominantly elastic. In the process of aging, or as a residual of injury, there is a relative increase in the percentage of fibrous elements. As the relative increase of fibrous elements occurs, the disc loses its elasticity, and its recoil hydraulic mechanism decreases. The "older" annulus reveals a replacement of the highly elastic collagen fibrils by large fibrotic bands of collagen tissue devoid of mucoid material. This disc is, therefore, less elastic.

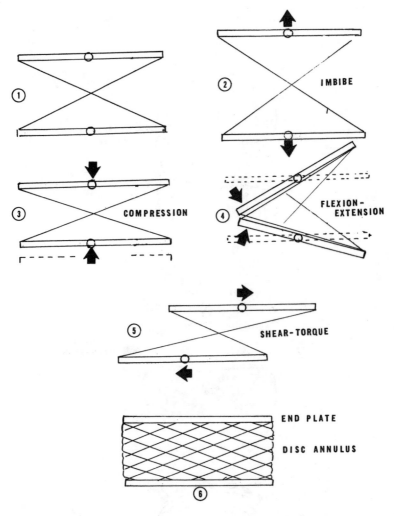

FIGURE 4. *1*. Annular fibers at rest. *2*. Effect of elongation. *3*. Effect of compression. *4*. Effect of flexion or extension. *5*. Effect of translatory torque.

The nucleus pulposus is a colloidal gel, a mucopolysaccharide that has a physical-chemical action. In a "young" and in an undamaged disc the nucleus is 88 percent water. Due to its colloidal chemical nature it can imbibe external fluids and maintain its intrinsic fluid balance. Diffusion of solutes occurs via the central portion of the end plates and through the annulus (Fig. 5). Increased intradiscal pressure probably also forces fluid through minute foramina in the end plates. When pressure is released or decreased, fluid returns into the disc by imbibition. As the nucleus ages, it loses its water-binding capacity. After the

5

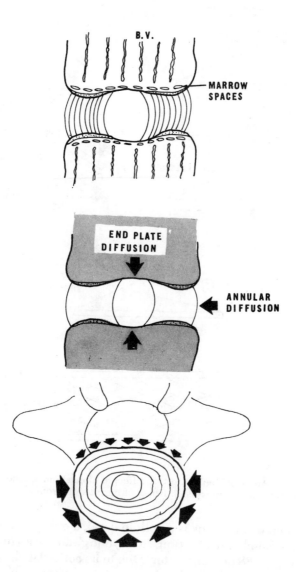

FIGURE 5. Disc nutrition through diffusion. Diffusion of solutes occurs through the central portion of the end plates and through the annulus. Marrow spaces exist between circulation and hyaline cartilage and are more numerous in the annulus than in the nucleus. Glucose and oxygen enter via the end plates. Sulfate to form glucosaminogly-cans enters through the annulus. There is less diffusion into the posterior annulus. (B.V. = blood vessels.)

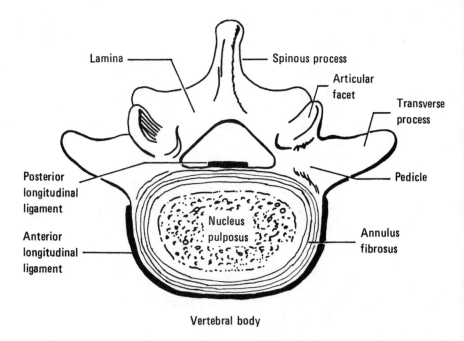

Lamina — — Spinous process

Articular facet

Transverse process

Posterior longitudinal ligament

Pedicle

Nucleus pulposus

Annulus fibrosus

Anterior longitudinal ligament

Vertebral body

FIGURE 6. Vertebral segment. As viewed from above, the vertebral segment is divided into the anterior and posterior segments. The anterior portion is the vertebral body and the disc structures. The posterior portion consists of the lamina, pedicles, and facets. In this segment the posterior longitudinal ligament is incomplete, placing it at the lower lumbar (L$_5$) level.

first two decades the nucleus water content decreases from its early 88 percent because its water-binding capacity has been decreased. In the aging process there is a decrease in the protein polysaccharide with an additional loss of osmotic and imbibition properties.

The intervertebral disc has a vascular supply that disappears after the second decade. By the third decade the disc, now avascular, receives its nutrition by diffusion of lymph through the vertebral end plates and by virtue of the physical-chemical imbibitory characteristics of the nucleus colloidal gel. The ability of an injured disc to regain its elasticity is bound to be stronger in the young.

Resistance to stress by the vertebral column is further augmented by the vertebral ligaments. The ligaments run longitudinally along the vertebral column and by their attachments restrict excessive movement of the unit in any direction and prevent any significant shearing action. The ligaments, by their position and attachments, encase the disc and reinforce the annulus yet do not detract from its physiologic elasticity. Viewed at the level of the functional unit, the entire disc is enclosed anteriorly by the anterior longitudinal ligament and posteriorly by the posterior longitudinal ligament (Fig. 6).

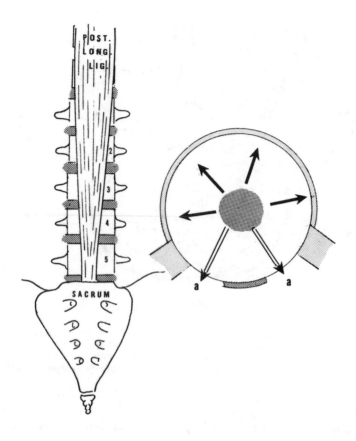

FIGURE 7. Diagrammatic sketch of posterior longitudinal ligamentous deficiency. The rear view drawing shows the narrowing of the ligament that begins at L_1. By the time it reaches L_5 it covers less than half the posterior disc margin. The double arrows in the small sketch show where disc herniation may bulge into the spinal canal.

Of functional and potential pathologic significance is the fact that the posterior longitudinal ligament is intact throughout the entire length of the vertebral column until in its caudal approach it reaches the lumbar region. At the first lumbar level (L_1) it begins to narrow progressively so that upon reaching the last lumbar (L_5) first sacral (S_1) interspace it has half of its original width. This ultimate narrow posterior ligamentous reinforcement contributes to an inherent structural weakness at the level where there is the greatest static stress and the greatest spinal movement producing the greatest kinetic strain (L_5-S_1) (Fig. 7).

Such is the anatomic construction of the anterior portion of the functional unit for its weight-bearing and shock-absorbing function. The

8

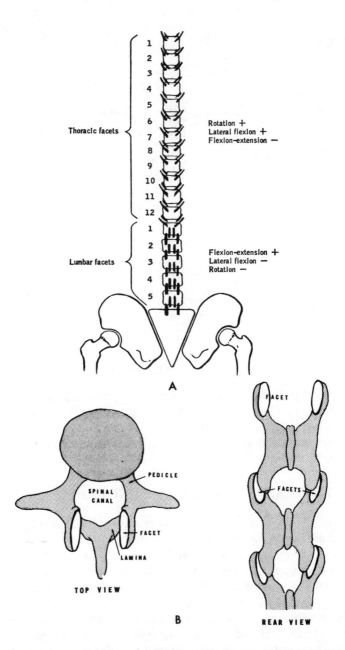

FIGURE 8. Direction of spinal movement is determined by the planes of the articular facets. A. The planes are vertical in the lumbar region, thus only anterior-posterior motion (flexion-extension) is possible in this region. Lateral bending and rotation are prevented. The plane of the thoracic facets permits rotation and lateral flexion but denies flexion and extension. The direction of movement permitted and prevented is indicated for the individual sections. Plus signs indicate possible motion; minus signs mean motion prevented. B. Details showing facets.

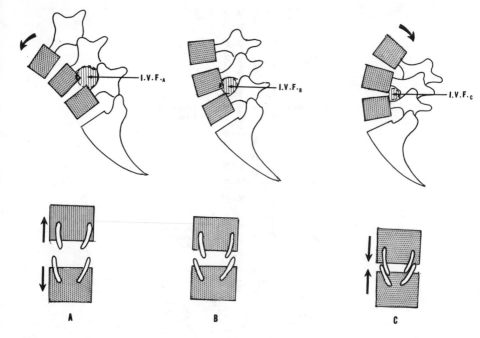

FIGURE 9.   Facet movement in flexion and hyperextension.

anterior portion of the functional unit is one of three "joints" contained in the total unit. The posterior portion of the functional unit containing the other two joints of the functional unit. In contrast to the anterior weight-bearing portion of the functional unit, the posterior portion has a guiding function.

POSTERIOR PORTION OF FUNCTIONAL UNIT

The posterior portion of the unit is composed of the two vertebral arches, two transverse processes, a central posterior spinous process, and paired articulations, inferior and superior, known as facets (Fig. 8).

The processes of the posterior arch, the transverse and the posterior spinous, are the sites of muscular attachment. Because of the origin and insertion of muscles from one process to another, movement of the spine is possible. Because of the contractility and the elasticity of the muscles, a large range of motion is possible, and the manner of attachment and interspinous bridging provides balance of the *static* spine and strength for the *kinetic* spinal column. Maintenance of the erect posture is in part achieved by the sustained tonus of the muscles acting on these bony prominences. Motion and locomotion are also dependent on these muscles playing synchronously between their points of bony attachment.

The articulations, or facets, pilot the direction of movement between two adjacent vertebrae. By their directional planes they simultaneously prevent or restrict movement in a direction contrary to the planes of the articulation. They may be compared to the movement of wheels on railroad tracks in which forward and backward movement is possible but sideway movement is prevented.

The facets are arthrodial joints that function on a gliding basis. Lined with synovial tissue, they are separated by synovial fluid which is contained within an articular capsule. The plane of the facets, in their relation to the plane of the entire spine, determines the direction in which the two vertebrae will move. The direction, or plane, of the facets in any segment of the spine will determine the direction of movement permitted to that specific segment of the spine. The plane of the facets will simultaneously determine the direction of movement not permitted that spinal segment. Movement contrary to the direction of the plane obviously is prevented or, at least, markedly restricted.

Because in the lumbar region the facet planes lie in the vertical sagittal plane, they permit flexion and extension of the spine. Bending forward and arching backward are thus possible in the lumbar region. Due to the vertical sagittal facet plane, significant lateral bending and rotation are not possible. The male portion of the facets fitting into the female guiding portion permits movement in the direction of the guides, but lateral, oblique, or torque movement is *mechanically prevented* in the lordotic posture. In a slightly forward flexed position or posture in which the lordosis is decreased, the facets separate, thus allowing movement in the lumbar area, in a lateral and rotatory direction (Fig. 9). In lumbar hyperextension the facets approximate, thus eliminating completely any lateral or rotatory movement.

In the thoracic spine the facets are convex-concave and lie essentially in a horizontal plane. Movement permitted by this facet plane in the thoracic spine is lateral flexion, such as side bending and rotation about a vertical line. A combined movement of lateral flexion and rotation occurs here, for, in spinal column movement, no pure lateral bending is possible without some rotation and no true rotation is possible without some lateral flexion. Due to this facet plane, no significant flexion or extension movement in an anterior posterior plane is possible in the adult thoracic-spine segment (Fig. 10).

In brief, the direction of the facet plane that exists between two adjacent vertebrae in a functional unit determines the direction of movement of those two vertebrae. As the facets of the lumbar spine are vertical-sagittal in an anterior plane, movement of the lumbar spine exists in an anterior-posterior flexion-extension direction. The planes of the thoracic spine relegate to this segment all significant lateral flexion such as side bending and rotation of the total spine. All other

11

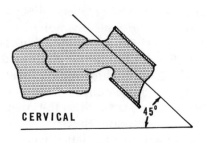

CERVICAL 45°

FIGURE 10. Angulation of planes of vertebral facets. The angulation that determines the direction of movement at various vertebral levels is depicted.

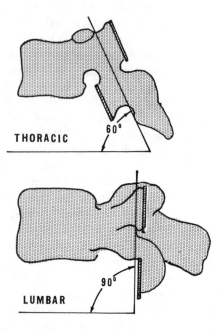

THORACIC 60°

LUMBAR 90°

significant movement is barred to these segments. In this generalization of total spinal movement the cervical spine segment is intentionally excluded.

TOTAL SPINE

The total vertebral column can now be visualized as the *sum total* of all the *functional units*, superimposed one upon the other, in an erect jointed column balanced against gravity and capable of movement. Having studied the functional anatomy of the individual functional unit, we can now study the total vertebral column from a static and a kinetic viewpoint.

The *static* spine as observed from the side has three basic physiologic curves. A fourth curve, that of the coccyx below the sacral

12

base, is a nonmobile inflexible curve with no pertinent effect upon man's attempt to maintain his balance in the erect position, and, therefore, its consideration is omitted in the study of the physiologic curves.

The entire spine is balanced on the sacrum, at its base, as a flexible segmented rod is balanced by a juggler. Immediately above the sacrum, the lowermost curve is the lumbar lordosis. This lordosis is convex anteriorly and forms its curve within a five vertebral body segment. The next curve, cephalad to the lumbar lordosis, is the thoracic curve which is termed the "dorsal kyphosis." The thoracic curve has its convexity posteriorly and being composed of 12 vertebrae has a curve of lesser curvature than is present in the lumbar curve. The bones of the thoracic vertebrae are smaller, and the discs are thinner, each disc being less pie-shaped than its comparative disc in the lumbar region. The cervical lordosis is the uppermost physiologic curve with an anterior convexity similar to the lumbar lordosis, and because of smaller vertebrae, thinner discs, and different bony configurations forms a smaller arc.

All three curves—the lumbar, the thoracic, and the cervical—in their ascent, must meet in a midline center of gravity to balance the weight distribution of the curve and to counter the eccentric loading of each curve. The side view of the three physiologic curves in the erect position may be considered as *posture* (Fig. 11).

The sacrum is the foundation platform upon which is balanced the superincumbent spinal column (Fig. 12). As the sacrum is firmly attached to both ilia, these bones move *en masse* as one unit, constituting the pelvis. The pelvis is centrally balanced on a transverse axis between two ball-bearing joints formed by the rounded femoral heads of the femors fitted into the cuplike acetabular sockets, which permit a rotatory motion in an anterior-posterior plane. By pivoting in a rotatory manner between these two lateral points, the pelvis may rotate back and forth, simultaneously rocking and changing the angle of the sacrum (Fig. 13).

Movement of the pelvis on its transverse axis constitutes "rotation" of the pelvis. Upward movement of the anterior pubic portion of the pelvis, termed "upward rotation," has the effect of lowering the sacrum with a decrease in the sacral angle. Downward movement of the front portion of the pelvis, called "tilting" of the pelvis, elevates the rear portion of the pelvis, changes the angle of the sacrum, and increases the sacral angle. The sacral angle is determined as the line drawn parallel to the superior border of the sacrum measured in relationship to a horizontal line. The plane upon which the lumbar curve is balanced and ascends is thus variable and can change in its inclination according to the relationship of the pelvis.

As the lumbar spine ascends upward at an angle perpendicular to the level of the sacral surface, the acute angle of the sacrum causes the

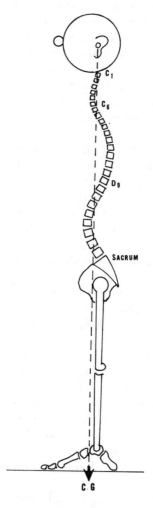

FIGURE 11. Posture. The physiologic curves of the erect vertebral column transect the center of gravity (CG) at the regions shown.

lumbar spine to arise at a slight vertical angle. Thus the lumbar spine needs only a slight degree of arching to return to midline. With an increase in the sacral angle, due to tilting of the pelvis, the plane of the sacrum becomes more obtuse, the lumbar spine takes off at a sharper angle to the horizontal and must, therefore, arc through a sharper curve to return to midline. The greater the sacral angle, the more angled the lumbar take-off demands that the curve which will bring the spine back into center of gravity balance must be even sharper. Those few words, "the greater must be the curve," specify essentially a greater *lordosis* of the lumbar spine.

In contrast a smaller angle brought about by elevating the pubic bone which depresses the sacrum, thereby decreasing the angle of the

14

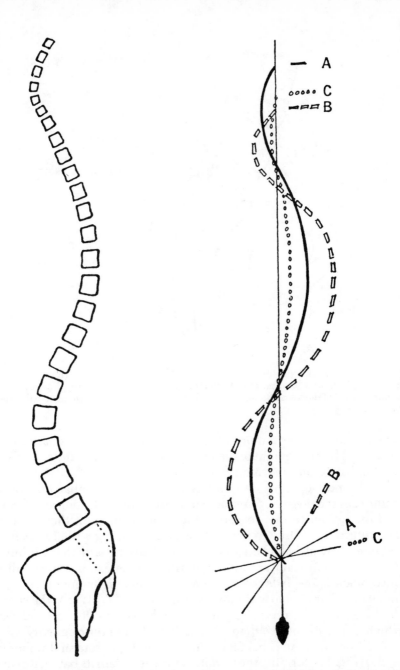

FIGURE 12. Static spine considered erect posture (relationship of physiologic curves to plumb line of gravity). *Left:* Lateral view of the upright spine with its static physiologic curves depicting posture. *Right:* The change in all superincumbent curves as influenced by change in the sacral base angle. All curves must be transected by the plumb line to remain gravity balanced. *A* is physiologic; *B*, increased angle; and *C*, decreased sacral angle with flattened lumbar lordosis.

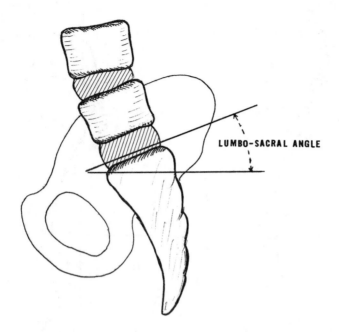

LUMBO-SACRAL ANGLE

FIGURE 13. Physiologic lumbosacral angle. The lumbosacral angle (LSA) is computed as the angle from a base parallel to horizontal and the hypotenuse drawn parallel to superior level of the sacral bone. The optimum physiologic lumbosacral is in the vicinity of 30 degrees.

sacral base, permits a more erect lumbar spine with a smaller arc, o. lordosis. This movement of the pelvis is called *tilting** and the effect on the lumbar lordosis termed *flattening*.

As the pelvic angle determines the angle of lumbar take-off and influences the degree of lumbar curvature so must the degree of lumbar lordosis influence the degree of the superincumbent thoracic curve. The return to midline to prevent eccentric loading will always force a flexible vertical balanced rod to curve back toward the midline. As there is insignificant anterior-posterior flexion-extension mobility of the thoracic spine, balance occurs as a rigid total segment moving at the thoracolumbar joint to maintain its equilibrium (T_{12}-L_1). At the summit, the balance of the remaining spine is achieved in the cervical region which balances the head and keeps it at the center of gravity.

The lumbar spine is balanced upon the oblique screen (lumbosacral angle) (Fig. 13), forming the *lordotic* curve to regain its balance over the center of gravity. The curve is so destined because of the shape of the

---

* "Tilting" (here employed to mean "to cause flattening of the lumbar lordosis") is used in a clinical sense, whereas functional anatomists use the term in an opposite sense to imply anterior elevation of the pelvis.

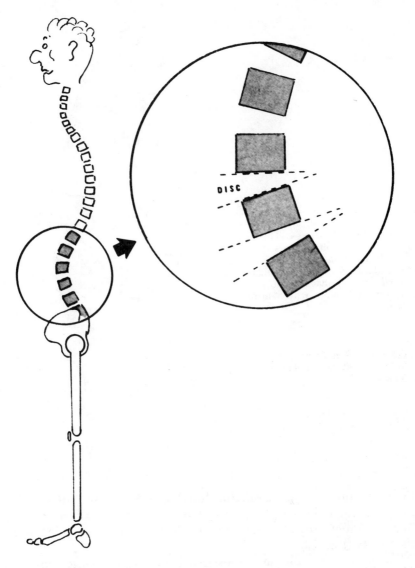

FIGURE 14. The physiologic curves are determined largely by the shape of the inter-vertebral discs (*insert*).

disc (Fig. 14), but there is a *shearing* stress upon the lower lumbar vertebrae.

Because of the short spinous processes of the functional units, the supraspinous ligament essentially passes behind the tips of the posterior-superior spine process. The ligamentous attachments of L_4 and L_5 minimize the forward shearing of these vertebrae (Fig. 15).

As the ligaments remain relatively relaxed in the full erect posture,

17

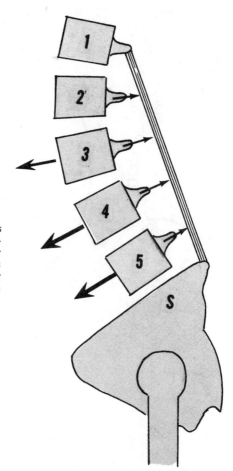

FIGURE 15. Shear stress. The lordosis of the lumbar spine causes the vertebrae to have an incline plane shear force (*large arrows*). The ligaments (*small arrows*) attach to the posterior spinous ligaments which minimize shearing.

the facets must assume a relationship that assists in minimizing shearing. Although the facets are not considered to "bear weight," this implies direct vertical weight-bearing, but tangential shear is borne by the facets (Fig. 16).

The three physiologic curves that comprise the *static* spine and designate *posture* are unequivocally influenced by the sacral angle. In other words, pelvic rotation is the mainstay of erect posture. Lateral viewing of the three curves of the nonmoving erect spine gives a true picture of the posture of the erect *adult*.

While one quarter of the adult spine is composed of disc material, the remaining three quarters consists of bony vertebrae. As the upper and lower vertebral cartilaginous plates are essentially parallel, the degree of curving is largely determined by the shape of the discs. If all the vertebrae were superimposed on each other without the interposition

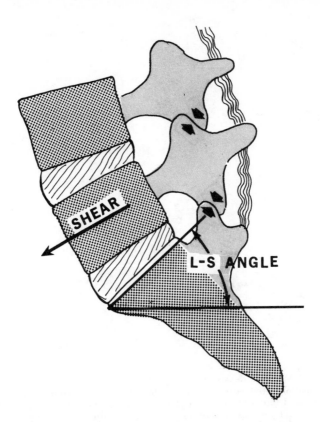

FIGURE 16. Shear stress on facets. Forward and downward shear of the fifth lumbar vertebra upon the sacrum is borne by the facet (*arrows*) when the longitudinal ligaments are lax.

of the intervertebral discs, the physiologic postural curves would not exist. The discless spine would form a very slight curve with its convexity posterior. The curve formed by the discless spine would resemble that of the newborn child. Development of the upright adult posture evolves in a chronological pattern from the first posture of the newborn.

The spine of the newborn has none of the adult physiologic curves, but instead has a total flexion curve of the curled-up infant *in utero*. The total curve is slightly more arched than is the ultimate adult thoracic kyphotic curve, and the curve is of similar convexity. There are no lordotic curves in the lumbar or cervical spinal areas of the newborn child.

During the first 6 to 8 weeks of life, the child raises his head and by this antigravity maneuver initiates the muscular action of the erector muscles that form the cervical lordosis. As crawling and sitting ultimately evolve, the lower lumbar spinal curve develops in an antigravity

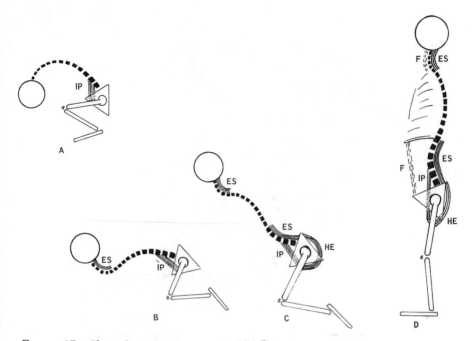

FIGURE 17. Chronologic development of posture. *A*. The total curve of the fetal spine *in utero*. *B*. Formation of the cerivcal lordosis when the head overcomes gravity. *C*. Formation of the second lordotic (lumbar) curve due to the antigravity force of the lumbar erector spinae (ES) muscles and the restriction of the iliopsoas muscles (IP). *D*. Erect adult posture showing the strong antigravity erector muscles (ES and HE hip extensors) and the weak flexor (F) muscles of the neck and abdomen.

action. The dorsal kyphosis has no antigravity influence even when an erect posture is reached, so that the change that evolves is merely a slight increase in its initial *in utero* convexity.

The addition of the two lordotic curves gives primarily the anti-gravity effect of the erector muscles which develop in the child as it attempts and finally achieves the upright-erect position. The lordotic curves originate partly from the original strength of the antigravity muscle and in some measure from the weakness of the opposite mus-culature, such as that which exists in the abdominal muscle and in the anterior neck-flexor muscles.

The lumbar lordosis is caused largely by the failure of the hip flexors to stretch and elongate. In the fetal position the hips and knees are flexed against the abdomen of the child in its "curled up in a ball" position. As the legs extend, the iliopsoas muscle elongates slowly but incompletely. The iliacus because of its influence upon the inner aspect of the ilium to the anterior-upper thigh acts to keep the hips flexed. The psoas originates from the anterior aspect of the lumbar

20

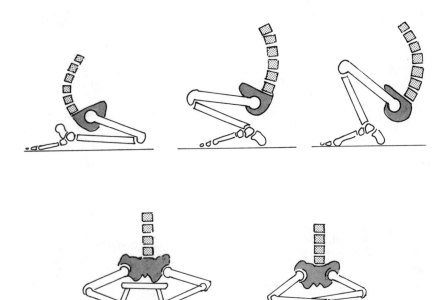

FIGURE 18. Sitting postures common to Eastern cultures.

spine and enters upon the anterior aspect of the femur. As the hips extend to assume the erect posture, extension at the hip joints causes a simultaneous forward traction on the lumbar spine via the psoas attachment, causing anterior convexity or lordosis (Fig. 17).

POSTURE

The upright adult exhibits balanced physiologic curves. Static spinal configuration can be considered "good posture" if it is an effortless, nonfatiguing posture, painless to the individual who can remain erect for reasonable periods of time, and present an aesthetically acceptable appearance.

These criteria of normalcy must be considered in ascertaining the cause of painful states and the factors demanding correction. Significant deviations from physiologic static spinal curves can cause discomfort and disability.

There are many factors that influence adult posture, but there are three factors that supersede all others in their prevalence and frequency. (1) Familial-hereditary postures, such as marked dorsal kyphotic spine, a noticeable "sway back," etc.; variations in ligamentous laxity, muscle tone, and even psychologic motor drive have a

21

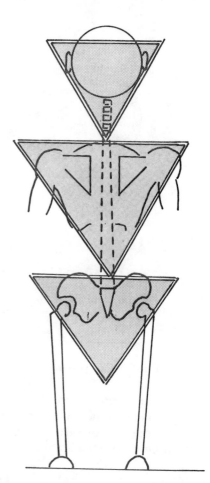

FIGURE 19. Body engineering of stance performed with broad, heavier parts at the top, situated upon a narrow base.

familial-hereditary component. (2) Structural abnormalities influence posture. Such abnormalities may be congenital or acquired, may be skeletal, muscular, or neurologic, and may be static or progressive. Postural defects can occur as the result of neuromuscular diseases, such as cerebral palsy, parkinsonism, and hemiplegia. The influence on the postural structures from diseases, such as rheumatoid arthritis and poliomyelitis, and from peripheral nerve injuries needs no elaboration. More insidious in its influence and admittedly more controversial in its acceptance is (3) the posture of habit and training.

Postural influences attributable to a familial or hereditary origin and postural deviations established by the external influences of neuromuscular, articular, or bony pathology can usually be established by correct history, complete physical examination, and specific laboratory and roentgen-ray studies. Many diseases portray a specific diagnostic picture that reveals the diagnosis at a glance. The influence of some diseases on posture may be less clearly defined, but further study of the effect of disease on posture can produce additional diagnostic tools.

The effect of habit or training on posture presents a study that has its own share of controversy and difference of opinion. Postural training in childhood by parental control or training by educators in our schools has a profound influence in laying the groundwork of ultimate adult posture. Posture is to a large degree habit and from training and repetition can become a subconscious habit. The subconscious habit of posture is manifested not only in static posture but to a large degree in kinetic patterns. Repetition of faulty action can result in faulty kinetic function and repeated faulty posture patterns can become ingrained.

The ordinary upright posture with arms hanging loosely at the side or clasped in front or behind is universal. Sitting in a chair is not. One quarter of the human race habitually takes weight off its feet by crouching in a deep squat at rest or at work (Fig. 18). Chairs, stools, and benches were in use in Egypt and Mesopotamia 5000 years ago, but the Chinese used chairs only as recently as 2000 years ago. Before that time they sat on the ground as do the Japanese and Koreans. The Islamic societies of the Middle East and North Africa have returned to sitting on the floor "for cultural prestige."

A deep squat position for work and rest is used by millions of people in Asia, Africa, and Latin America. The Turkish or "tailor" cross-legged squat is used in the Middle East and India and in much of Asia. The practice of crossing the legs or folding them to one side, which was thought to be assumed by women because of narrow skirts, is found in cultures where clothing is not worn.

Standing is influenced by the use of footwear as well as a complex of many factors: anatomic, physiologic, cultural, environmental, occupational, technologic, and sexual.

Of interest is the cultural attitude toward posture. Religious concepts have influenced posture by prescribing periods of kneeling, bowing, standing, and prostration during worship. Western postural codes have been relaxed in the course of the past century. Eighteenth-century chairs with hard seats and straight backs have been replaced by soft curved chairs or sofas. We still, however, train our children to conform to cultural norms of posture by verbal instruction.

Standard posture is one of skeletal alignment refined as a relative arrangement of the parts of the body in a state of balance that protects the supporting structures of the body against injury or progressive deformity. This was the definition given by the Posture Committee of the American Academy of Orthopaedic Surgery in 1947.

The body is poorly engineered for standing because stance is maintained with the heavy parts at the top upon a narrow base (Fig. 19).

23

Balance is more efficient with less energy expenditure if none of the parts is too far from the vertical axis.

Posture must also be viewed from the cultural aspects of training, background, and childhood environment. Parental example is of undoubted significance in the establishment of accepted normal posture. Competition and example from siblings or classmates will also leave its mark on the psyche which in turn molds the postural patterns.

Posture to a large degree is also a somatic depiction of the inner emotions. There is no doubt that posture can be considered a somatization of the psyche. We stand and we move as we feel. Our stance and our movements mirror clearly to the observer our psychologic inner drives or their absence. Consciously or unconsciously we assume a pose to portray our inner feelings, and we move in a manner that depicts our attitude toward ourselves, our fellow man, and our environment. Our posture is "organ language," a feeling-expression, in fact a postural exteriorization of our inner feelings.

The depressed, dejected person will stand in a "drooped" postural manner with the upper back rounded and the shoulders depressed by the "weight of the world carried on his back." This is the familiar bodily expression when one is too tired to "stand any more of this." Such posture is a picture of fatigue and becomes in itself a fatiguing posture. The posture of fatigue places a chronic ligamentous strain upon an individual and the muscular effort exerted to relieve the strain may be too feeble to be effectual.

The hyperactive hyperkinetic person will portray his feelings in posture as well as in the abruptness and irregularity of his movements. The movements of alertness need not be, and in fact usually are not, those of efficiency and effectiveness. This posture depicts that of the uneasy aggressor, in combat pose, ready to leap or ready to withdraw in a defensive crouch. In observing this type of person, the doctor need not ask his psychologic attitude but should merely observe his sitting, standing, walking, response to questions, and movements during the interview and examination.

The tall girl may stand slumped. In childhood she wished to be shorter as were her companions. She stooped "down to their height." Her counterpart, the short girl, stood "to her full height" to be taller, by standing on her toes, with her head erect, her chest protruding and her low back arched. The full-bosomed girl, influenced by teasing or fearing to lack modesty, sat, stood, and walked with rounded shoulders to decrease the apparent size of her bosom.

All patterns of posture assumed in childhood for real or imagined results form a pattern that becomes deep seated. The pattern becomes not only a psychic pattern, but it gradually molds the tissues into somatic patterns that remain a structural monument to early psychic molding. When the age of "reason" or realization is reached the posture is largely fixed in its structural composition and is deeply established in the subconscious. Without extreme persistent effort to change, that posture will become a permanent fixture.

Feldenkrais[1] states that improper head balance is rare in young children except in structural abnormalities. However, repeated emotional upheavals cause the child to adopt attitudes that ensure safety. This, he claims, evokes contraction of the flexor muscles inhibiting extensor tone. His analogy to animals is that when they are frightened they react by violent contraction of all flexor muscles, thus preventing (inhibiting) the extensor musculature. This prevents running or walking. A similar reaction occurs in newborns as a reaction to the fear of falling.

The attitude of the child from repeated emotional stresses is that of flexion with concurrent inhibition of the extensors. This attitude in the upright erect posture becomes one of flexion at the hips and spine with a forward head posture. This posture becomes habitual and feels "normal."

The pain-causing postural pattern can be ascertained by understanding the deviation from what is considered normal. A full evaluation of the mechanisms of pain production in the *static* then in the *kinetic* spines will follow, but the exact sites of pain production must first be determined. When the site of tissue capable of eliciting pain can be located, the specific movement or positions of the vertebral components that irritate these tissues can be established. For the evaluation of the sites in the vertebral column capable of painful reaction we must return to the *functional unit* (Fig. 20).

TISSUE SITES OF PAIN ORIGIN

The intervertebral disc itself is a non-pain-sensitive tissue. The total disc is an inert tissue and the nucleus has been found completely free of any sensory type of nerve endings. Nerve endings have been found in the annulus, but neurophysiologic studies have failed to discover pain sensory transmission from these nerves. The discs, therefore, both annulus and nucleus, must be considered insensitive to pain sensations.[2,3,4]

If the absence of sensory nerves emanating from the disc be accepted it must be assumed that it is not possible to consider the disc a pain-producing unit. The commonplace disc-pain must, therefore, originate from contiguous tissues, with the disc itself in some manner participating in the instigation of disc-pain by its action on these surrounding tissues.

If the internal pressure within a normal disc is experimentally in-

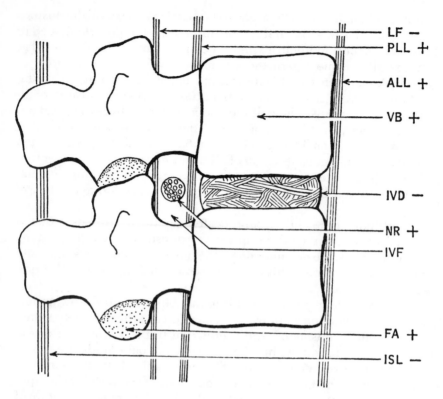

FIGURE 20. Pain-sensitive tissues of the functional unit. The tissues labeled + are pain-sensitive in that they contain sensory nerve endings that are capable of causing pain when irritated. Tissues labeled – are devoid of sensory nerve endings.

IVF = intervertebral foramen containing nerve root (NR).
 LF = ligamentum flavum
PLL = posterior longitudinal ligament
ALL = anterior longitudinal ligament
IVD = annulus fibrosus of intervertebral disc
 FA = facet articular cartilage
ISL = interspinous ligament

creased by injecting saline solution into the disc the mere increase of such pressure does not cause pain. In a disc, however, that has previously been degenerated, which degeneration can be considered fragmentation of the annulus with a dehydrated nucleus, increase in the interdiscal pressure causes an ache in the region of the low back.[5]

If the same method of increasing pressure within a disc of known degeneration is used no pain sensation occurs when the posterior longitudinal ligament is anesthetized by procaine. It can be assumed then that the irritation of the posterior longitudinal ligament by increase in internal pressure within a degenerated disc is the mechanism

26

of pain production, and the posterior longitudinal ligament is the pain-sensitive tissue. The posterior longitudinal ligament therefore must contain sensory nerve endings.

It is apparent that a normal disc has sufficient elasticity and resiliency to withstand significant increases in internal pressure which will prevent a bulging irritation of contiguous tissues. Degeneration of a disc due to annular fragmentation decreases its resiliency and resistance to increase in internal pressure, permitting encroachment on surrounding tissues.

The ligamentum flavum and the interspinous ligaments are nonsensitive.[6] Similarly, stimulation or movement of the dura mater elicits no sensation of pain. These tissues, therefore, must be classified as insensitive to pain.

The synovial lining of the facets and the articular capsule of these joints are richly supplied by sensory as well as vasomotor nerves. The synovial tissues of these joint spaces respond to stimuli and inflammations as do all other synovial joint tissues elsewhere in the body. Inflammatory responses of these tissues result in swelling and engorgement of the synovial linings, increase viscosity of the synovial fluid, causing periarticular muscle spasm that results in progressive limitation of movement. The part becomes "frozen" or at least significantly immobilized. Inflammation of synovial joints produces dull to severe pain depending on the severity and extent of the inflammation.

The concomitant muscle spasm that accompanies spine dysfunction is in itself capable of eliciting pain. In animal experiments, painful irritation of the lumbosacral joints and ligaments causes reflex spasm of the erector spinae and hamstring muscles. This spasm in a human being undoubtedly is painful. In addition to pain resulting from the joint and ligamentous irritation, there can arise irritation from the sustained muscle spasm, compression of the interposed intervertebral disc by the spasm of the muscle, which will result in pain if any disc degeneration exists. In the presence of any disc degeneration the spasm can constitute a significant compressive force. Multiple factors, such as these, can be seen to contribute to the production of pain at the functional unit level.

Another factor is the sciatic nerve root which emerges through the intervertebral foramen. It is a combined motor-sensory nerve and thus is a pain-sensitive nerve. Irritation of this nerve evokes pain localized to the dermatome distribution of the specific rootlet irritated.

Pain elicited from irritation of the nerve root, felt either locally or distally, is considered as resulting from dural irritation. The dura is innervated by the recurrent nerve of Luschka (Fig. 21).

As the nerve roots descend the spinal canal, they cross the disc immediately above the foramen. The roots enter the foramina beneath

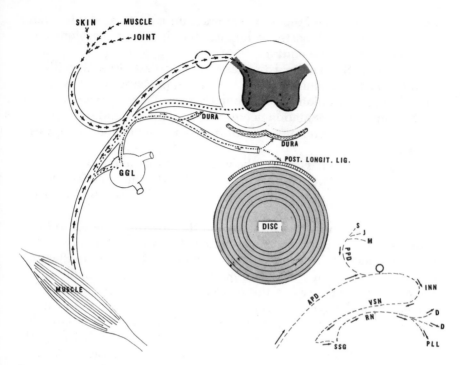

FIGURE 21. Innervation of the recurrent nerve of Luschka.

PPD – posterior primary division
APD – anterior primary division
GGL – sympathetic ganglion
INN – internuncial neurons
VSN – ventral sensory nerve
SSG – sensory sympathetic ganglion
 RN – recurrent nerve of Luschka
  D – to dura
PLL – posterior longitudinal ligament

the pedicle. After they leave the foramina, they incline downward, outward, and *forward.* In the lower disc levels the nerves enter the origin of the psoas muscle (Fig. 22). By virtue of their vertical entry into the foramen, they are located in the superior aspect of that foramen (Fig. 23).

At their entry into the foramen on their extravertebral course, they invaginate the dura and the arachnoid and carry a sheath of each *into* the foramen. The arachnoid continues along the nerve root as far as the ganglion (Fig. 24). The dura continues along the combined nerve (sensory and motor portion) until it fuses with the arachnoid, forming the distal end of the sleeve. The dura then continues along the distal nerve, forming the outer fibrous sheath of the nerve, the perineureum.

The posterior (sensory) nerve root is twice the thickness of the an-

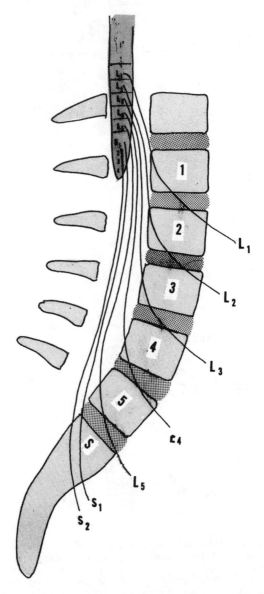

FIGURE 22. Relationship of nerve roots to vertebral levels.

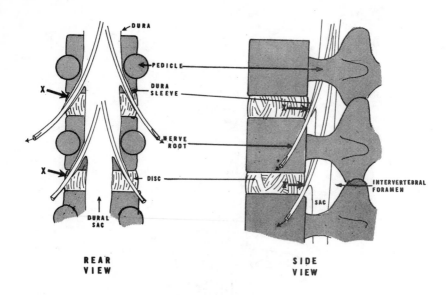

REAR
VIEW

SIDE
VIEW

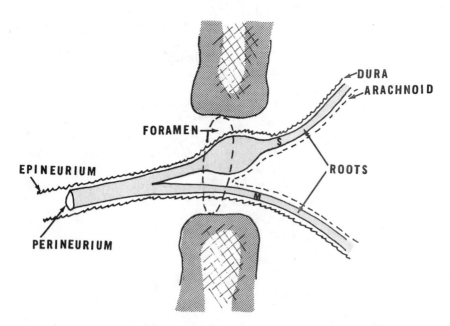

FORAMEN

EPINEURIUM

PERINEURIUM

DURA
ARACHNOID

ROOTS

FIGURE 24. Dural and arachnoid sheaths of the nerve root complex. The arachnoid follows the sensory and motor nerve roots to the beginning of the intervertebral foramen and follows the sensory root to the beginning of the ganglion. The dura follows the nerve roots until they become the combined sensory and motor nerve outside the foramen and continues as the perineurium and epineurium. Neither the dura nor the arachnoid attaches to the intervertebral foramen.

30

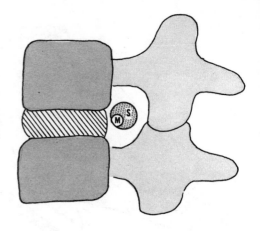

FIGURE 25. Sensorimotor aspect of nerve root. Within the intervertebral foramen the motor roots are smaller than the sensory and are inferior and posterior near the disc.

terior (motor) root. These remain separate until encountering the ganglion of the sensory root, at which point they merge into a single funiculus. In their further descent and outward migration the motor nerve roots are concentrated anterioinferiorly in the funiculus (Fig. 25).

The nerve roots and their dural sleeves are attached loosely to the foramina and are permitted to move. The nerve axons have plasticity, but the dura has no elasticity. Traction distally or dorsally pulls the entire nerve fiber-dura complex in either direction. The nerve roots intrinsically elongate, whereas the dura increases in tension. This will be discussed further in the chapter on disc herniation.

Within the foramen the nerve and its sheath occupies 35 to 50 percent of the space. The remainder of the foramen is filled with loose areolar connective tissue, adipose tissue, arteries, veins, lymphatics, and the recurrent nerve of Luschka (Fig. 26).

Upon emergence from the foramen, the nerves divide into their anterior and posterior primary division, sending immediately a branch to the facet joints (Fig. 27). Within the foramen only the dura innervated by the recurrent nerve of Luschka is apparently pain-sensitive. The posterior longitudinal ligament also innervated by this nerve is likewise sensitive.

We have ascertained which tissues within the functional unit are capable of eliciting pain, and we have depicted the static erect spine by combining and superimposing the functional units. Now we must make our upright person move and, in moving, the normal must be established so that deviations capable of causing pain can be understood.

LIGAMENTOUS-MUSCULAR SUPPORT

Consideration of the periarticular tissues and muscular influence on the kinetic spine involves once again a discussion of the static spine

31

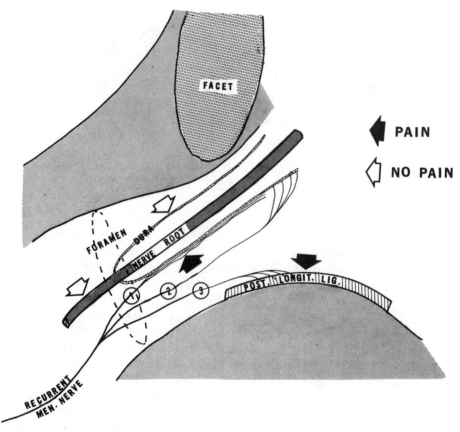

FigURE 26. Dura accompanying nerve root through intervertebral foramen with its innervation by the recurrent meningeal nerve. 1 and 2 proceed to the anterior dural sheath, illustrating the sensitivity of that portion of the dura. The posterior dural sheath with no innervation is insensitive. 3. Innervation which is capable of pain supplies the posterolongitudinal ligament.

because a balanced erect static spine requires minimal muscular effort.

Physiologic erect balance is essentially a ligamentous function relieved by intermittent small muscular contractions that are triggered by proprioceptive reflexes of the joints and ligaments. The muscles of an erect but relaxed man are electromyographically silent except for those in the gastrocnemius groups. The calf muscles which balance the leg at the ankle joint are the only continually active muscular group affecting posture.

Ligamentous support is effortless and thus not fatiguing. Excessive or prolonged ligamentous stress is relieved by muscular contraction and, as muscular effort is fatiguing, is held to a minimum for economy of energy expenditure. Good posture requires balance between

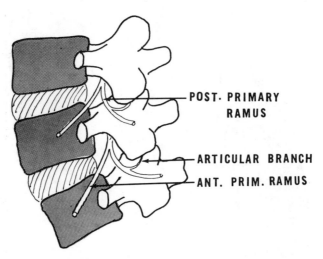

POST· PRIMARY
RAMUS

ARTICULAR BRANCH

ANT. PRIM. RAMUS

FIGURE 27. Division of nerve roots. Upon emergence from the foramen, the roots divide into the anterior primary division and the posterior primary division. A small articular branch is sensory to the facets.

ligamentous support and minimal, yet adequate, muscle tone. Improper posture or prolonged stress from awkward positions causes protracted ligamentous strain resulting in discomfort. Strain may arise because of muscular fatigue which no longer affords ligamentous relief.

For proper posture, the static spine is dependent on the pelvic angle. The pelvis is held in ligamentous balance by the anterior hip joint and the "Y" ligament. This "Y" ligament, the iliopectineal ligament, is a fibrous reinforcement of the anterior portion of the hip joint that prevents hyperextension of the hip. In erect stance, man "leans forward on this ligament."

The knee joint can similarly be "locked" in extension when it relies on the posterior popliteal tissue that prevents overextending the knees. This position eliminates the need for any muscular effort on the part of the quadriceps femoris. The lumbar spine can "lean" on the anterior-longitudinal ligament and the abdominal wall. The ankle joint, however, cannot be "locked" in any position so that muscular effort is required constantly.

The pelvis is further supported by the tensor fascia latae. These fascial bands mechanically assist the "Y" ligaments as well as limit lateral shift of the pelvis. Their course from the iliac crests downward and backward to insert at the iliotibial band at the knee lends itself well to reinforcing the "Y" ligament and helps lock the knee (Fig. 28).

The pelvic angle is the key to ligamentous posture. Rotation of the pelvis will initiate a total unlocking of all the balancing joints and necessitate muscular effort.

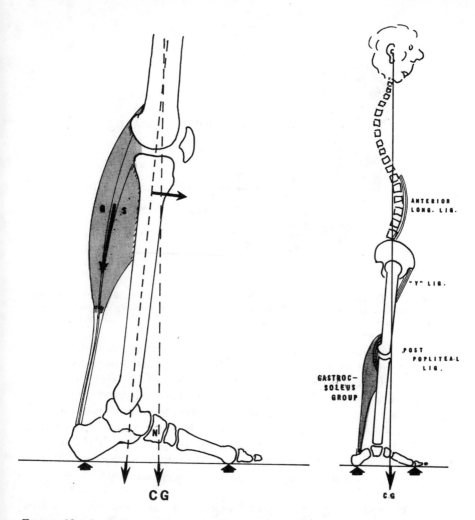

ANTERIOR
LONG. LIG.

"Y" LIG.

POST
POPLITEAL
LIG.

GASTROC—
SOLEUS
GROUP

C G

C.G

FIGURE 28. Static spine support. The relaxed person leans on his ligaments: the iliofemoral ligament, ("Y" ligament of Bigelow), the anterior longitudinal ligament, and the posterior knee ligaments. The ankle cannot be "locked," but by leaning forward only a few degrees the gastrocnemius must contract to support the entire body. Relaxed erect posture is principally ligamentous with only the gastroc-soleus muscle group active.

To study the erect person functioning in anterior-posterior plane, it is best to view him from the rear because it will then be possible to see the deviations from the normal in their relation to an imaginary vertical line.

The upright supporting beams of the pelvic floor are the legs, and if the parallel legs are equal in length the supported platform will be horizontal. If the tibia and femurs of both legs are in direct alignment and of equal length, the femoral heads must be equidistant from the ground, and the transverse axis through the femoral heads must be

34

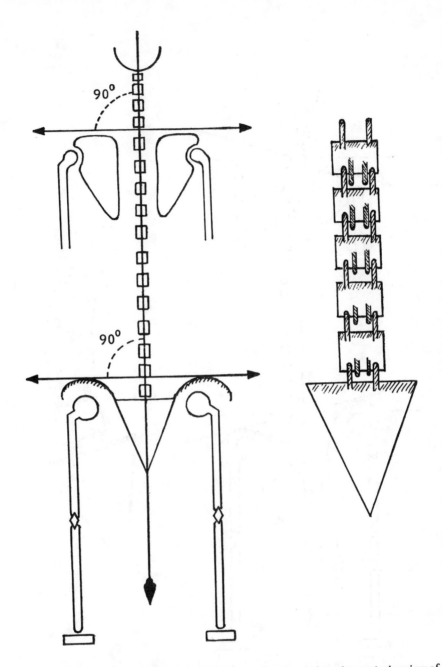

FIGURE 29. Spinal alignment from anterior-posterior aspect. Anterior-posterior view of the erect human spine. With both legs equal in length the spine supports the pelvis in a level horizontal plane and the spine, taking off at a right (90-degree) angle, ascends in a straight line. The facets shown in the enlarged drawing on the right show their parallel alignment and proper symmetry in this erect position.

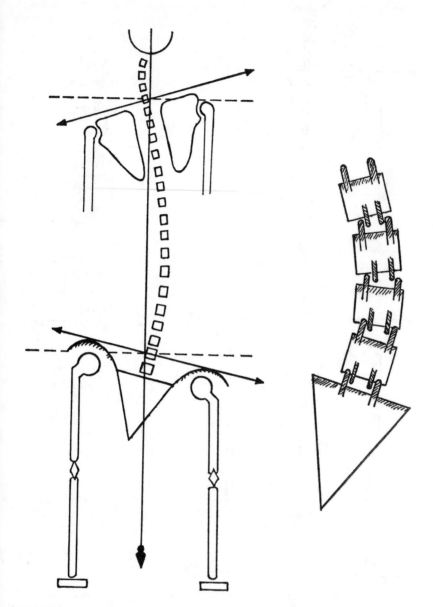

FIGURE 30. Pelvic obliquity and its relationship to spinal alignment. Anterior view of an oblique pelvis due to a leg-length discrepancy. Owing to pelvic slant in a lateral plane, the spinal take-off is at a lateral angle. The flexible spine will curve in an attempt to compensate, and the facets of the curving spine will become asymmetrical in relationship to each other.

horizontal. Balanced between these two points the pelvis will rotate around a level axis.

In the static spine a level pelvis viewed from behind will reveal the spine ascending from the pelvic base at right angles and so continuing cephalad will find the head perched in direct mid-line over the center of the sacral point (Fig. 29). This head-pelvic center relationship obviously presupposes a straight spine.

A structurally straight spine of adequate flexibility will permit symmetrical bilateral side-bending. When we recall that lateral spine movement occurs in the thoracic region and not in the lumbar area, an equal degree of bending to the left or to the right will demand that the midpoint be level. This action requires a truly vertical lumbar spine. Symmetry in the act of side-bending requires lateral flexibility of the spine. As no significant lateral bending occurs in the lumbar spine the angle of take-off from the lumbar spine at the pelvic level will determine the amount of correction the dorsal spine must take to effect a return to the center of gravity.

Another important factor is leg-length discrepancy which will cause a pelvic obliquity. The causes of leg-length differences are numerous. A unilateral *genu valgum* or unilateral *genu recurvatum* will cause the side involved to be of shorter length. A unilateral leg-length discrepancy can result from fractures, articular disease, amputation per se or from an improperly fitted prosthesis. Childhood diseases (such as osteochondrosis, poliomyelitis, and hip dysplasia), that may impair unilateral leg growth, can lead to unequal leg lengths in adult life. The effect of leg-length difference on the pelvic level has an apparent influence on the static spine when it is seen from the anterior-posterior position, and the obliquity of the pelvis has an equal effect on the kinetic spine (Fig. 30).

KINETIC ASPECT OF TOTAL SPINE

The total erect spine that has been described in its static postural state is capable of movement and now must be analyzed in its kinetic potentialities. The functional units are the component operational units of the entire spinal column and, as the units individually move, so moves the total column.

Movement is initiated by muscular action exerting its traction effect through its muscular attachments upon the bony prominences of the functional unit. A constant attempt is made by the antigravity forces to maintain balance against gravity. Of these antigravity forces, muscular action initiated by a proprioceptively stimulated righting reflex immediately attempts to correct the "off-center" shift. During movement, the body makes a constant effort to maintain its balance.

Movement of the total spine has been previously pictured as that of an articulated flexible rod requiring movement at each component segment. Movement at the anterior portion of the functional unit is permitted by the fluid shift of the nucleus pulposus within its elastic annulus. Excessive movement is prevented by fascia and the longitudinal ligaments which, by their resiliency, exert a cushioning effect and thus protect the fibers of the annulus from bearing the full tearing effect of forceful flexion or excessive extension.

The facets have been ascribed as the guiding portion of the functional unit permitting flexion-extension in the lumbar region and rotation lateral-flexion in the thoracic area because of the directional plane of the facet joints. All movement contrary to this articular plane is essentially prevented.

The extent of the permitted range of motion is thus determined by the extensibility of the longitudinal ligaments, the elasticity of the articular capsule, the fluidity of the disc, and the elasticity of the muscles. Since it is known that direction of movement of the lumbar spine is the effect of flexion and extension, it may be asked to what extent these movements are possible in the normal spine.

Extension of the lumbar spine may be slight, but it is usually possible to a moderate degree. Most children have the capability of arching backwards to a large degree, and with training and persistent exercise this function may persist through adulthood. Inherited ligamentous laxity will enhance this more extreme hyperextension. The anterior longitudinal ligament plays the major restricting role in limiting hyperextension.

Forward flexion of the lumbar spine is possible to a much smaller extent than is extension. Such forward flexion of the lumbar spine is possible *only* to the *extent of and slightly more* than the *reversal* of the static lumbar *lordosis* (Fig. 31).

The lumbar spine, which is usually composed of five vertebrae, must have its movement occur within the five intervertebral interspaces. In total flexion the degree of flexion movement varies at each interspace. Most forward flexion movement occurs at the last interspace which is the intervertebral space between the last lumbar (L_5) and the sacrum (S_1). An estimated three quarters (75 percent) of all lumbar flexion occurs at this interspace, which marks the junction of the lumbar spine to the sacral-pelvic bone and constitutes the *lumbosacral joint.*

Owing to the absence of flexion in the thoracic spine and with the postulation that 75 percent of lumbar flexion occurs at the lumbosacral joint, it may be argued then that 75 percent of all spine flexion occurs at the lumbosacral joint and at L_4-L_5.

The remaining percentage of forward flexion is proportioned between the remainder of the lumbar-vertebral interspaces. Fifteen to 20

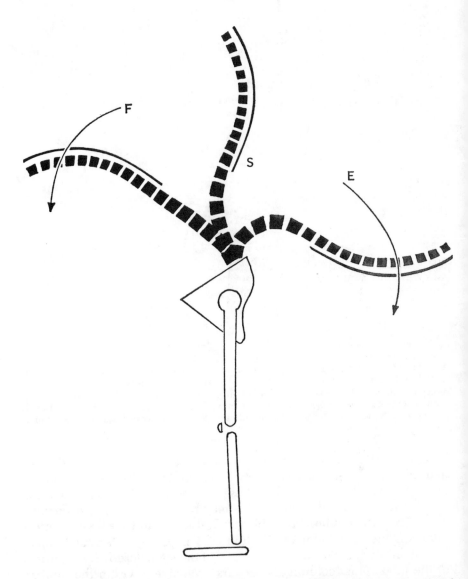

FIGURE 31.   Flexion-extension of total spine. Composite diagram depicting flexion and extension of total spine. Flexion of the lumbar spine occurs to the extent of reversing slightly past the lordosis, whereas extension is moderate. In all movements of flexion, extension, or static erect position the thoracic spine does not alter its curve. (F = flexion; S = static spine; E = extension.)

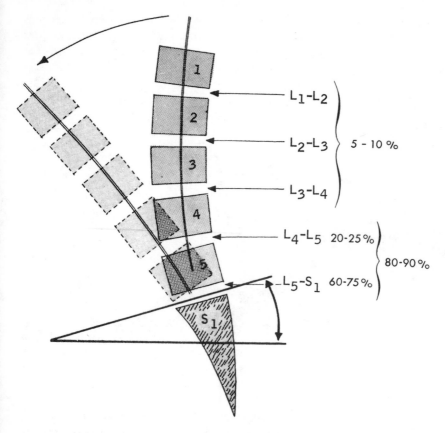

FIGURE 32. Segmental site and degree of lumbar spine flexion. The degree of flexion noted in the lumbar spine as a percentage of total spine flexion is indicated. The major portion of flexion (75 percent) occurs at the lumbosacral joint; 15 to 20 percent of flexion occurs at the L_4-L_5 interspace; and the remaining 5 to 10 percent is distributed between L_1 and L_4. The forward-flexed diagram indicates the mere reversal past lordosis of total flexion of the lumbar curve.

percent of flexion occurs between L_4 and L_5 vertebrae, and the remaining 5 or 10 percent occurs between L_1 and L_4. The greatest portion of this last 5 to 10 percent of flexion is found between L_2 and L_4 (Fig. 32).

The theory of *total* trunk *flexion* may be summarized as occurring primarily at the lumbosacral joint, the L_4-L_5 joint and to a lesser degree between the remainder of the lumbar vertebrae with total lumbar flexion limited to the extent of reversal of the static lordosis. Extension of the total spinal column also occurs exclusively within the lumbar segment but to a greater degree than the extent of flexion. No significant flexion-extension occurs in the dorsal spine.

If a person were to bend forward in an attempt to touch his fingers to the floor without bending at the knees, he would require more than the degree of flexion attributed to the lumbar spine flexion. Were this lumbar curve reversal the only flexion possible for the individual, less than half the distance toward the floor would be reached. Additional bending must be possible, and this flexion occurs at the hip joints.

The flexion possible at the hips is attributed to rotation of the pelvis around the fulcrum of the two lateral hip joints. Such rotation occurs in an anterior-posterior sagittal plane with the anterior portion or symphysis pubis area lowering or rising, while the sacrum at the posterior end of the rocker describes the same arc. The level of the sacrum changes its angle in respect to the horizontal as does a balanced teeter board.

As the pelvis rotates forward, the sacral angle becomes more obtuse, and the lumbar spines takes off at a more forward ascent. If no flexion of the lumbar spine had taken place when full forward rotation of the pelvis had occurred, the person may have been able to bend forward to a significant degree with his fingers almost touching the floor if his hips were sufficiently limber to permit that degree of pelvic rotation.

Smooth symmetrical total bending, however, is the result of the physiologic manner in which man is intended to bend. This is done with pelvic rotation and flexion of the spine occurring simultaneously. A smooth-graded ratio must exist between the degree of pelvic rotation and the degree of lumbar lordotic reversal that constitutes the *lumbar-pelvic rhythm*. The mathematical relationship of lumbar curve, or the lordosis, and reversal to the simultaneous degree of rotation of the pelvis, which is the change in the sacral angle, constitutes the fundamental *kinetic* concept of the spine. This rhythmic relationship of spine-trunk-flexion to pelvic rotation is similar in body mechanics to the *scapulohumeral rhythm* considered to be the physiologic *kinetic* pattern of the shoulder girdle.

EXTENSOR MUSCLES OF THE SPINE

The erector spinae (sacrospinalis) originates from the last two thoracic vertebrae, all the lumbar vertebrae, the sacral spines, the sacrum, sacroiliac ligament, and all the medial aspect of the iliac crest. Below the twelfth rib the muscle splits into three columns:

1. iliocostal—lateral band,
2. longissimus—intermediate band,
3. spinalis—medial band.

The iliocostal (lateral) inserts into the angle of the ribs and ultimately extends to C_{4-6}. In the thoracic spine the muscle extends over six segments (ribs).

41

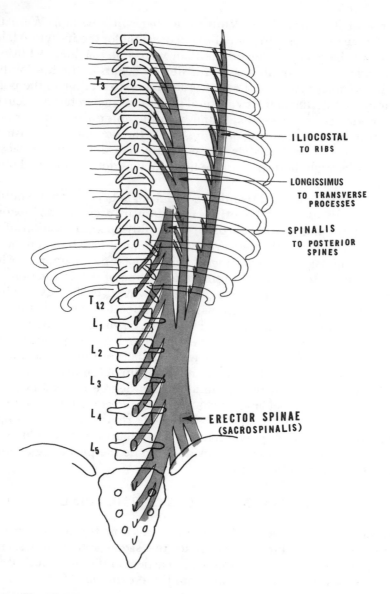

ILIOCOSTAL
TO RIBS

LONGISSIMUS
TO TRANSVERSE
PROCESSES

SPINALIS
TO POSTERIOR
SPINES

ERECTOR SPINAE
(SACROSPINALIS)

FIGURE 33. The extensor muscles of the spine.

The longissimus (intermediate) inserts into the transverse processes cephalad to T_1. It is the only erector spinae muscle that reaches the skull.

The spinalis is essentially a *flat aponeurosis*. Its medial border attaches to the posterior spines of the thoracic vertebrae. The lateral margin is free.

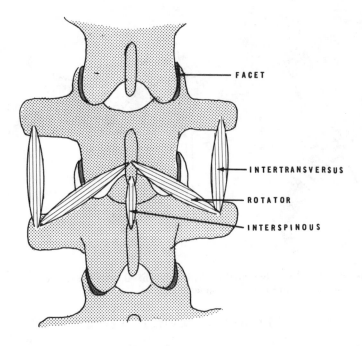

FACET

INTERTRANSVERSUS

ROTATOR

INTERSPINOUS

FIGURE 34. Deep extensor spinal muscles.

Under the erector spinae muscle is located the transverse spinalis which comprises three layers:

1. semispinalis,
2. multifidus,
3. rotatores.

The semispinalis (superficial layer) arises from the tips of the transverse processes and inserts into the tips of the spinous process. It spans 3 to 5 segments (Fig. 33).

The multifidus arises as a thick, fleshy mass on the dorsum of the sacrum (between the spinous and transverse crest), from the overlying erector spinae aponeurosis, and from *all* the transverse processes up to C_4. This muscle spans three segments to attach to the inferior border.

The rotators spans one segment: from the transverse process of one vertebra to the spinous process of the adjacent vertebra (Fig. 34).

In the lumbar spine there are other small muscles: (1) interspinalis unite adjacent lumbar spinous processes, and (2) intertransversari unite adjacent transverse processes.

The thoracolumbar fascia is the dorsal aponeurosis of the transversus abdominal muscles.

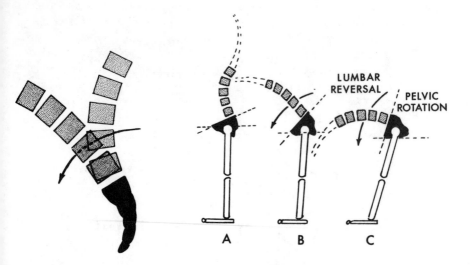

FIGURE 35. Lumbar pelvic rhythm. With pelvis fixed, flexion-extension of the lumbar spine occurs mostly in the lower segments L_{4-5} and L_5-S_1.

LUMBAR-PELVIC RHYTHM

The lumbar-pelvic rhythm (Fig. 35) can be perceived as the ratio between two movements occurring simultaneously in one plane. Reversal of the lumbar curve is difficult to grade in a numerical formula that would be simple, clear, and concise. The *lumbar* portion of the rhythm is initially a flattening, then a gradual reversal of an arc that was not originally a perfect sphere. The lumbar curve does not reverse equally at all points along its sphere. The difference of movement at the L_5-S_1 segment compared to the movement between L_2-L_3 indicates the irregularity of the arc as it flattens out and reverses. Nevertheless, there is significant smoothness of curve change to correlate it in a smooth kinetic relationship with a simultaneous secondary movement of pelvic rotation.

During the change of lumbar curve from concave to flat, to convex, occurs the secondary movement of pelvic rotation. The *pelvic* phase of the rhythm is merely the rotation of the pelvis around the transverse axis of the two hip joints. Pelvic rotation, in total spinal flexion, is rotation of the pelvis starting with the sacral angle as noted in the *static* spine, followed by a smooth gradual increase of the angle as the anterior portion of the pelvis descends and the posterior aspect ascends. The sacral angle which increases in flexion decreases in extension as the body returns to the erect *static* stance. The grading of this rotation is easy to calibrate mathematically as the movement consists merely of rotation around a central point.

Lumbar-pelvic rhythm is a simultaneous movement in a rhythmic ratio of a lumbar movement to a pelvic rotation, the sum-total-movement consisting in the person's bending forward and returning to an erect position. At any phase of total body flexion the extent of lumbar curve flattening must be accompanied by a proportionate degree of pelvic rotation. When complete body flexion has been attained, the lumbar curve must have fully straightened and reversed, thus presenting a lumbar convexity while the pelvis must have rotated to the full extent permitted by the hip joints. The rhythm is so smooth and precise that at every point in the process there will be equality between lumbar reversal and pelvic rotation.

In forward flexion most of the spinal flexion occurs by the time the trunk is inclined 45 degrees forward. The remainder of forward flexion occurs as a rotation of the pelvis. In resuming the erect posture the opposite movement occurs.

The lumbar disc, being of equal thickness anteriorly and posteriorly, allows as much flexion as extension from the position of rest, except that in the lower lumbar region the disc is thicker anteriorly than posteriorly, thus allowing *less* flexion than extension.

In forward flexion the lumbar joints flex as the extensor muscles lower the body weight above the lowest lumbar joint. By 45 degrees of flexion, the tension in the ligaments has increased and that in the muscles decreased[7-10] (Fig. 36). Further flexion occurs as a rotation of the pelvis by relaxation of the posterior leg and hip muscles when the pelvis relaxes.

In lifting a heavy object (or the reverse, in lowering a heavy object), the pelvis at first rotates with the ligaments of the lumbar spine bearing the brunt of the stress until 45 degrees of flexion is reached, at which point the muscles of the back become active (Fig. 37).

One of the mechanical advantages of flexing the hips and knees is that it places the hip extensors at a mechanical advantage. Another advantage is that the quadriceps femoris group assists in the lifting and simultaneously tenses the iliotibial band which is the site of attachment of the glutei. By flexing the hips and knees, the distance between the weight being lifted and the center of gravity is decreased[11] (Fig. 38). As the spine flexes, the shoulder girdle and the pelvis (hip joint) comes closer together, which decreases the lever arm for lifting (Fig. 39).

In the discussion of the lumbar-pelvic rhythm the emphasis has been on *flexion,* but the exact converse of the thythm must occur in the return to erect position after flexion. It is obvious that return from any point must begin at a concise point in the rhythm at some place during the descent. Just as every point in the lumbar flexion must be matched by a concise point in the degree of pelvic rotational tilting so must return to the erect be synchronously perfect. Full return to upright

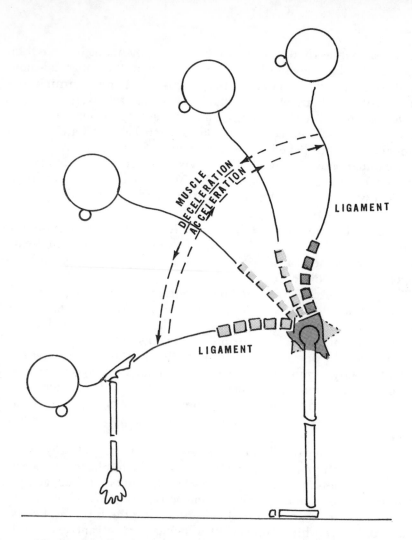

FIGURE 36. Muscular deceleration and acceleration of the forward-flexing spine from the erect ligamentous support to the fully flexed ligamentous restriction. Muscle eccentric and concentric contraction permits forward flexion and re-extension.

finds the pelvis derotated to its more acute lumbosacral angle while the lumbar curve resumes its erect static lordosis (Fig. 36 in reverse).

Man in his action of bending forward and straightening up must conform to accurate smooth lumbar-pelvic rhythm which, being kinetic, is a neuromuscular pattern of action as well as a mechanical function. This neuromuscular pattern is partly acquired and partly inherited. Deviation, however, can occur, and faulty habit can be learned and repeated until the deviation becomes a deep-seated habit pattern. Proper rhythm similarly can be perfected by learning and acquired habits.

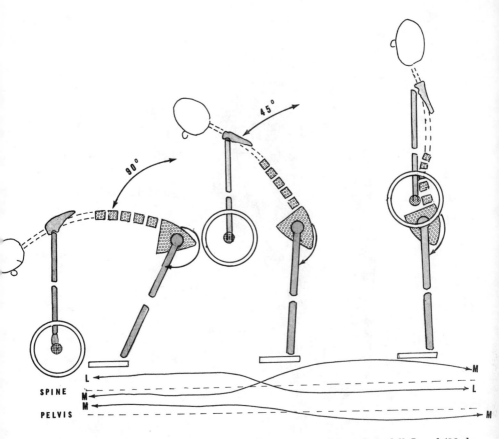

FIGURE 37. Muscle-ligamentous control in lifting. In lifting from full flexed (90 degrees) to half erect (45 degrees), the lumbar spine is supported by its ligaments (L) with posterior pelvic muscles (M) bearing the stress effort. From 45 degrees of flexion to full erect the spine extensor muscles contract and complete the full extension.

The neuromuscular pattern must be precise and work together with faultless mechanical action of the spine. All the moving parts must be unimpeded. As any defective part in an otherwise integrated machine will impair total function so will inadequacy of any of the component parts of the lumbar-pelvic mechanism destroy proper rhythm.

Reference to component parts again draws attention to the functional unit. Adequacy of the unit demands competent discs. Anatomically symmetrical facets are necessary to permit accurate gliding, and the synovial linings of the articular surfaces must present no impediment to smooth motion.

The longitudinal ligaments the main function of which is limitation of motion must in turn permit sufficient and free movement existing throughout the length of the ligament. Segmental limitation in the

47

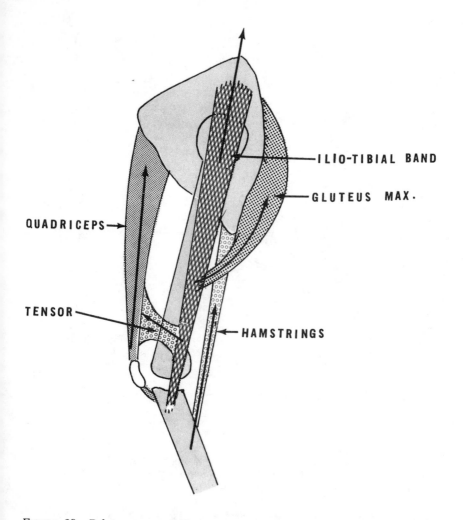

FIGURE 38.   Pelvic extensor mechanism. By flexing the knees, the quadriceps tense the iliotibial band to which is attached the glutei. This combination strengthens the pelvic rotation which extends the back in lifting.

elongation of any one ligament would cause excessive movement in the other less restricted segments. Limited elongation of the entire length of the longitudinal ligament would totally impair the lumbar phase of the rhythm. Physiologic spine flexion requires resiliency for the posterior longitudinal ligament while the paraspinous muscles must have equal elasticity.

Pelvic rotation is directly dependent on the adequacy of the hip joints to rotate fully in a ball-bearing manner. This requires a normal hip-joint socket working bilaterally. The intactness of the joint socket must be

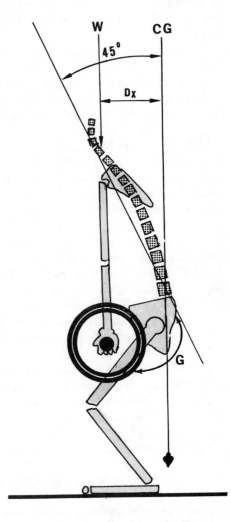

FIGURE 39. Mechanical advantage in lifting an object close to the body from 45 degrees to erect. The erector spinae muscles extend the spine upon the pelvis and "do the lifting." The shorter the distance of the weight (D_X) to the center of gravity (CG), the more efficient is the lever arm. The pelvis is rotated by the glutei (G), which are aided by the quadriceps and tensor band.

accompanied by resilient periarticular tissues and good muscular control of hip function. The third phase of the lumbar-pelvic rhythm in which the pelvic joint alters its relationship to the center of gravity also demands symmetrical integrity of the hip joints.

FACET PLANES

In the lumbar spine the facets are vertically parallel and their proper alignment demands a straight line. A curve in the lumbar spine will displace the relationship of the facets. The spinal curve of the structural scoliosis portrays vividly this imbalance. A curvature similar to this

49

structural scoliosis may exist merely because an otherwise flexible spine is affected by a pelvic obliquity caused by differential in leg length.

When the spine is straight and the facets symmetrical the articular surfaces glide without friction. If the facets deviate in their direction of movement, the articulating surfaces are no longer parallel, and friction or impingement may occur at some point in flexion-extension. In this respect the scoliosis resulting from a short leg does not differ markedly from a structural scoliosis.

Unilateral impairment of movement of any of the joints participating in the total movement of the lumbar-pelvic rhythm can cause asymmetry in flexion or extension. A hip joint that is damaged and will not rotate fully will prevent full rotation of the pelvis around its axis. Axis rotation is hindered at one end of its bilateral supports. One of the pair of ball-bearing joints "binds" in its rotation and thus places excessive strain at the other end. An extra-articular restriction of the joint, such as tight hamstrings on one side, can cause a similar asymmetrical restriction. The *lumbar-pelvic rhythm* becomes impeded by a unilateral defective part and the two halves of the body, left and right, perform the rhythm unequally. Furthermore, a fused ankle, by impeding the third phase of the rhythm, the posterior shift of the pelvis, has its adverse influence on the total rhythmic cycle.

Intrinsic structural facet asymmetry within an otherwise straight spine can adversely influence the rhythm. This asymmetry must be confirmed by x-ray studies and cannot be determined exclusively on clinical observation. As the total pelvic-lumbar rhythm mechanism requires all the component parts to function without hindrance, any break in continuity, any "weak link in the chain," will ultimately result in overall stress and the eventual breakdown of pain-free motion.

THORACOLUMBAR JUNCTION

It is well accepted that flexion-extension occurs in the lumbar spine by virtue of the sagittal plane of the facets[12-14] and that the thoracic spine flexes laterally with simultaneous rotation also by virtue of its facetal plane.[15,16] There is a less known or recognized rotation that occurs at the transition of the thoracic and lumbar spinal segments (T_{12}-L_1). As the superior facets of the twelfth thoracic vertebra are of the thoracic angulation and thus permit rotation and lateral flexion, the inferior facets are similar to the lumbar spine and permit only flexion and extension.

The thoracic spine is limited in rotation and lateral flexion by the intercostal tissues. Thus the thoracic spine moves essentially *en masse* as one segment. Most rotatory movement must therefore occur at T_{11}-T_{12}. Interspace studies[17] have revealed that approximately 90 degrees of rotation occurs between L_1 and L_5, 6 degrees rotation between the lower thoracic vertebrae, and 10 degrees at the thoracolumbar junction.

SUMMARY

The human spine is an articulated flexible structure composed of superimposed *functional units;* it is clear then that the total function of the spine depends on the integrity of each component part. The total functional unit is divided into two segments. The anterior portion is a hydraulic weight-bearing, shock-absorbing structure composed of two vertebrae and their interposed disc. The posterior section contains the articulating facets and functions as a guiding mechanism without weight-bearing facets.

The total spine comprises three physiologic curves which are formed by the shape of the intervening disc and in the lumbar segment forms a "lordosis," in the dorsal spine a "kyphosis," and in the cervical spine another "lordosis." These three curves transect the plumb line of gravity in order to remain in a state of balance.

Because the plane of the facets directs the movement of the spine at each segment, movement in a direction contrary to the facet plane is prevented. Vertical position of the lumbar facets determines anterior-posterior movement in a sagittal direction. Horizontal concave articular placement in the thoracic spinal segment places lateral bending and rotation of the total spine at this section.

The entire spine is balanced on an undulating pelvic base. The sacral portion of the pelvis by changing angle influences the superincumbent curves and thereby determines the *static* posture. Static stance is a ligamentously supported position requiring minimal muscular action.

The *kinetic* spine flexes and extends in a pattern of *lumbar-pelvic rhythm.* Smooth movement of the rhythm demands good neuromuscular integration, adequate flexibility of tissues, and competence of the participating joints.

Pain results from irritation or inflammation of pain-sensitive tissues within the functional unit. Improper static or inappropriate kinetic function can cause a painful reaction.

The appreciation of normal function is necessary before a true evaluation and interpretation can be made of the dysfunction in the causation of low back pain.

REFERENCES

1. Feldenkrais, M.: Body and Mature Behavior. International Universities Press, New York, 1975.
2. Roofe, P.G.: Innervation of annulus fibrosus and posterior longitudinal ligament. Arch. Neurol. Psychiatry 44:100, 1940.

51

3. Hirsch, C., Inglemark, B.E., and Miller, M.: The anatomical basis for low back pain. Studies on the presence of sensory nerve endings in ligamentous, capsular, and intervertebral disc structures in the human lumbar spine. Acta Orthop. Scand. 1:33, 1963-64.
4. von Luschka, H.: Die Nerven des menschlichen Wirbelkanales. H. Laupp, Tübingen, 1850.
5. Hirsch, C.: An attempt to diagnose the level of a disc lesion clinically by disc puncture. Acta Orthop. Scand. 18:132-140, 1948.
6. Stillwell, D.L.: The nerve supply of the vertebral column and its associated structures in the monkey. Anat. Rec. 125(2):139-167, 1956.
7. Farfan, H.F.: Muscular mechanism of the lumbar spine and the position of power and efficiency. Orthop. Clin. North Am. 6:135-144, 1975.
8. Farfan, H.F., and Lamy, C.: A mathematical model of the soft tissue mechanisms of the lumbar spine, in Buerger, A.A., and Tabis, J.S. (eds.): Approaches to the Validation of Manipulation Therapy. Charles C Thomas, Springfield, Ill., 1977.
9. Gracovetsky, S., Farfan, H.F., and Lamy, C.: A mathematical model of the lumbar spine using an optimized system to control muscles and ligaments. Orthop. Clin. North Am. 8:135-153, 1977.
10. Floyd, W.F., and Silver, P.H.F.: The function of the erector spinae muscle in certain movements and postures in man. J. Physiol. 129:184-203, 1955.
11. Farfan, H.F.: The biomechanical advantage of lordosis and hip extension for upright activity. Spine 3(4):336-342, 1978.
12. Wiles, P.: Movement of the lumbar vertebrae during flexion and extension. Proc. R. Soc. Med. 28:647-652, 1935.
13. Tanz, S.S.: To-and-fro range at the fourth and fifth lumbar interspace. J. Mt. Sinai Hosp. 16:303-307, 1950.
14. Allbrook, D.: Movements of the lumbar spine column. J. Bone Joint Surg. 39-B:339-345, 1957.
15. Arkin, A.M.: The mechanism of rotation in combination with lateral deviation in the normal spine. J. Bone Joint Surg. 32-A:180-188, 1950.
16. Roaf, R.: Rotation movements of the spine with special reference to scoliosis. J. Bone Joint Surg. 40-B:312-332, 1958.
17. Gregerson, G.G., and Lucas, D.B.: Axial rotation of the human thoracolumbar spine. J. Bone Joint Surg. 49-A(2): 247-262, 1967.

BIBLIOGRAPHY

Asmussen, E.: The weight-carrying function of the spine. Acta Orthop. Scand. 1(4):276-288, 1960.
Edgar, M.A., and Nundy, S.: Innervation of the spinal dura mater. J. Neurol. Neurosurg. Psychiatry 29:530-534, 1966.
Hendry, N.G.C.: The hydration of the nucleus pulposus and its relation to intervertebral disc dehydration. J. Bone Joint Surg. 40-B:132-144, 1958.
Hirsch, C., and Lewin, T.: Lumbosacral synovial joints in flexion-extension. Acta Orthop. Scand. 39:303-311, 1968.
Kaplan, E.B.: Recurrent meningeal branch of the spinal nerves. Bull. Hosp. Joint Diseases 8:108-109, 1947.
Splithoff, C.A.: Lumbosacral junction. J.A.M.A. 152:1610-1613.
Steindler, A.: Kinesiology of the Human Body. Charles C Thomas, Springfield, Ill., 1955.

CHAPTER 2

Abnormal Deviation of Spinal Function as a Pain Factor

To know the normal and to recognize the deviation from normal; to be able to reproduce the pain by reproducing the abnormal position or movement; and to understand the mechanism by which the pain is caused—this is the formula for the clinical evaluation of the patient with low back pain.

The spine functioning in a proper static and kinetic manner should not elicit pain. The presence of pain indicates irritation of a pain-sensitive tissue at some point in the functional unit or in its adjacent tissues. Irritation of these tissues implies dysfunction of the spine, either from the *static* or the *kinetic* aspect.

LUMBOSACRAL ANGLE—STATIC SPINE

In the static spine the vast majority of painful states can be attributed to an increase in the lumbosacral angle with a consequent accentuation of the lumbar lordosis. This increase in the lumbar lordosis is commonly termed "sway back." It is a safe assumption to credit 75 percent of all static or postural low back pains to such lordosis.

The lumbosacral angle is formed when the horizontal base of the angle is parallel to the ground level and the hypotenuse of the angle is formed at the level of the superior border of the sacrum (Fig. 40). The plane of the sacrum forms the base from which the lumbar spine takes off in its ascent and by which it achieves its balanced state.

The fifth lumbar vertebra lies upon the sacrum as a box rests on an inclined plane. The friction of the box on the incline, dependent on the weight of the box, prevents sliding, but there is the possibility of a sliding action down the incline plane which may constitute a shearing stress. As the angle of the sacrum increases, so does the slant of the inclined plane; thus the greater is the shearing stress (Fig. 41). Mathematically, an angle of 30 degrees will find the shearing stress to be 50

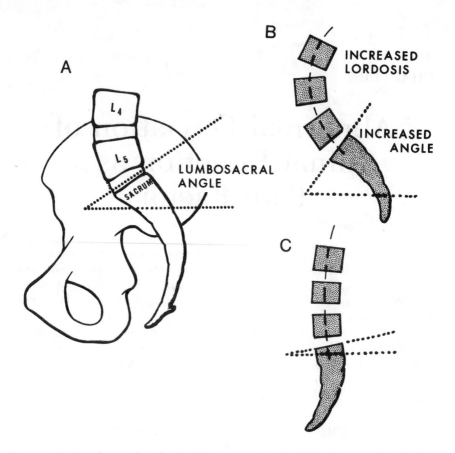

FIGURE 40. Lumbosacral angle. A. Erect posture angle. B. With increased angle the lumbar lordosis is increased. C. The lordosis decreases with decrease of lumbosacral angle.

percent of the superincumbent weight. An increase in the angle to 40 degrees will increase the shearing stress to 65 percent of the superincumbent weight. An angle of 50 degrees causes a shearing stress of approximately 75 percent of the weight of the movable object.

Increase of the sacral angle not only increases the degree of shearing stress at the lumbosacral joint but by changing the angle of the base influences the curvature of the lordotic curve. The greater the angle of the take-off base, the greater is the curve of the superincumbent spine, insofar as the lumbar curve (lordosis) must always return to the plumb-line center and must do so within five vertebral segments. A more acute angle of the sacral base forms a less sharply curved lumbar spine because the lumbar spine is then in more vertical position.

The degree of sacral angle influences the degree of angle of the fifth lumbar vertebra as computed to the horizontal base line. The shearing

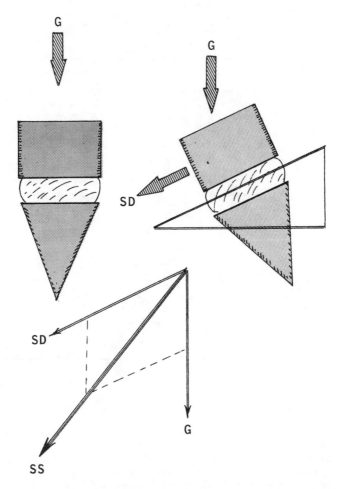

FIGURE 41. Static shearing stress of the last lumbar vertebra in its inclined plane relationship to the sacral vertebra. G implies the gravity stress of the entire body upon the weight-bearing hydraulic system of the intervertebral disc. SD is the force of a body sliding down an inclined plane. SS represents the resultant force and its direction of G and SD and is the shearing stress exerted on the elastic fibers of the annulus.

stress is proportional to the angle of the sacral inclination. The degree of angulation of the fourth vertebra on the fifth, the third on the fourth, the second on the third, decreases as the angle immediately below is decreased. The shearing stress correspondingly decreases proportionately with each successive ascending vertebral segment as the angle of inclination approaches the horizontal (Fig. 42). At the third lumbar vertebra the inclined plane, upon which it rests, is formed by the superior margin of the fourth lumbar vertebra and is almost hori-

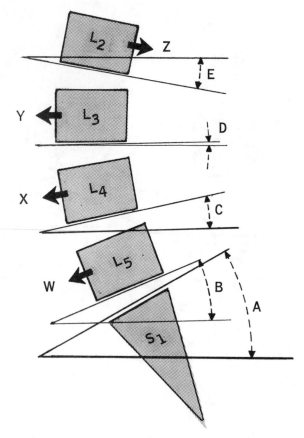

FIGURE 42. Differential shearing stress of lumbar vertebrae. The shearing stress of the last lumbar vertebra upon the first sacral differs from the shearing stresses of each successive cephalad vertebra. At each intervertebral level the inclined plane angle decreases and thus the shearing stress and its direction decrease.

zontal; consequently there is only minimal tendency for the superimposed vertebra to slide forward and no shearing stress exists.

The anterior longitudinal ligament limits the extension of the lumbar spine. By its anterior attachment the opening of the intervertebral spaces is restricted. Any further attempt at extending the spine in this area results in closure of the posterior disc space (Fig. 43). Approximation of the posterior aspects of the vertebral bodies simultaneously approximates the posterior articulations.

When approximation of the posterior articulations causes a gliding of the facets into each other, they become weight-bearing units. Weight-bearing is not a physiologic function. When this occurs, the joint surfaces are compressed and synovial inflammation may result. Synovial inflammation is a pain-producing situation.

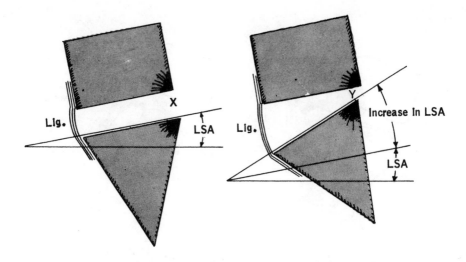

FIGURE 43. Mechanical analysis of posterior closure of the disc space by increase of the lumbosacral angle (LSA), anterior restriction of the anterior longitudinal ligament (Lig.). Narrowing of space X to space Y also portends approximation of the facets in their posterior relationship of the functional unit.

Besides the increase in lordosis that results from increase in sacral angulation, the increase in the incline causes greater shearing stress and places the facets in a position of "braking" action on the gliding superimposed vertebrae. This braking effort further compresses the articular synovial linings.

The so-called sway-back posture is one of relaxation in which the person leans forward on his "Y" ligament while the pelvis shifts anterior to the center of gravity. The front portion of the pelvis cannot rotate upwards because of the restriction of the "Y" ligament; thus the sacral angle increases. The lumbar spine must curve back toward the center of gravity and does so by increasing its curvature. Thus the posture of "relaxation" is also a stance of ligamentous strain.

The first steps of the infant are characterized by marked lumbar lordosis. This posture is in part due to the failure of the iliopsoas muscles to elongate as the hips extend which failure places traction on the lumbar spine. It is also accentuated by weak hip-extensor and weak abdominal muscles. These latter factors play a part in the posture of the elderly or of the middle aged who are not in condition and whose posture may be described as slovenly.

The painful low back of pregnancy is related to an increase in lordosis. The gravid uterus causes a slight shift forward of the pelvis as it does also in the relaxed pose. Besides, there is a fatigue during pregnancy that deters good habits and efforts in addition to a hormonal ligamentous laxity that completes the picture.

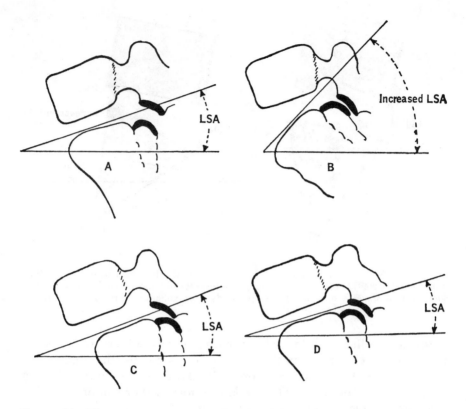

FIGURE 44. Variations in posterior articular relationships. A. Normal lumbosacral angle with intact disc: normal relationship of articular facets. B. Increase in lumbosacral angle (LSA) with posterior closure of the facets. C. Spondylolisthesis with a normal LSA exerting traction on the posterior longitudinal ligament and disruption of facet alignment. D. Disc degeneration with narrowing of intervertebral space and approximation of facets.

The condition of "kissing spines" is described in which the posterior superior spines actually contact as the result of increased lordosis and its concomitant posterior joint approximation. The contact of the posterior spines and accompanying irritation cause a pseudoarthrosis to form. This condition, known as the syndrome of Baastrup, which occurs in patients under 25 years of age, finds the pain reduplicated by hyperextension of the spine. A pseudoarthrosis can be observed on x-ray.

Increase in the sacral angle will initiate or intensify the pain of spondylolysis and spondylolisthesis, a full consideration of which is given in Chapter 5. Various mechanisms of posterior articular derangement are pictured in Figure 44.

Pain which derives from increased lordosis because of approximation of the posterior segment in the functional unit has been attributed in part to facet impingement and irritation. Posterior articular ap-

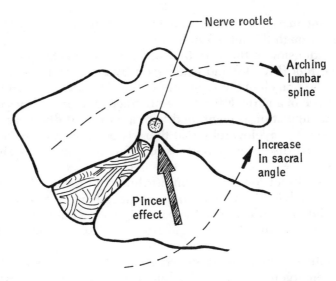

FIGURE 45. Nerve root impingement due to hyperextension of the lumbosacral spine. Greater extent of impingement can be expected with a degenerated disc.

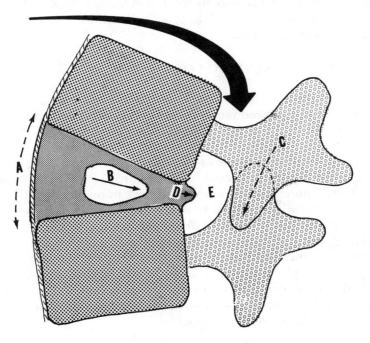

FIGURE 46. Disc protrusion in lumbosacral hyperextension. The anterior longitudinal ligament restricts further extension (A). The nucleus has deformed to the maximum, cannot migrate further anteriorly, and thus moves posteriorly (B). This causes a "bulge" (D) with encroachment into the intervertebral foramen (E). The facets overlap (C), which also narrows the foramen as well as causing painful weight-bearing.

proachment may also cause pain by irritating the nerve root as it emerges through the intervertebral foramen.

Hyperextension of the vertebral segment can mechanically irritate the nerve root (Fig. 45) and cause pain by compression of the main nerve or the branch of the recurrent nerve. This reaction can occur in the presence of a normal disc but with much greater facility when the increased angulation is combined with a narrowed disc space. It has been shown by myelography that there is posterior protrusion of the intervertebral disc from hypertension. This mechanism is shown in Figure 46.

The majority of low back pain attributed to posture is related to increase in pelvic tilt, increase in lumbosacral angle, concomitant increase in lumbar lordosis, and the pain originating from irritation of the facet synovial tissue. Contact and friction of the posterior superior spines causing low back pain must also be part of the evaluation, but this is relatively a rare condition. Irritation of the nerve root at its site of foramen emergence is possible, but in this condition the resultant pain more likely would manifest itself in the dermatome distribution rather than as a pain exclusively located in the low back region. Irritation of the recurrent nerve and the synchronous muscle spasm will refer pain to the low back area.

KINETIC LOW BACK PAIN

Pain caused by movement of the lumbar spine implies either a defective spine with impaired mechanical kinetics or a structurally normal spine functioning improperly. Kinetic pain implies irritation of pain-sensitive tissues activated by movements of the spine.

Pain may originate in the area of spine in one of *three* basic manners: (1) abnormal strain on a normal back; (2) normal stress on an abnormal back; and (3) normal stress on a normal back unprepared for the stress. The word *normal* as applied to strain implies a stress of reasonable magnitude that can be handled under average conditions without discomfort. A "normal" back refers to a structurally sound and functionally apt lumbar spine. The term normal, as always, has a relative value.

A good example of abnormal stress would be that of a person who suddenly has to catch a falling weight of several hundred pounds. Such an act would constitute an excessive stress that would overwhelm the muscles and ligaments of a normal back.

Abnormal Strain on Normal Back

A normal back, by the combination of muscle contraction which reduces the strain of the ligamentous structure, can sustain a superim-

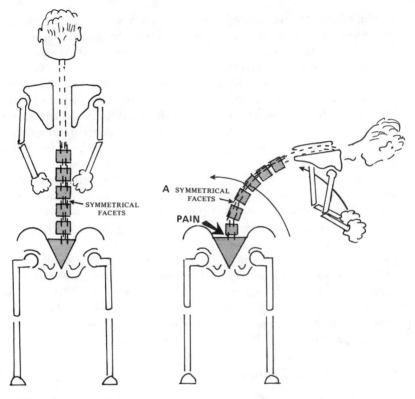

FIGURE 47. Asymmetrical facets. Pain can occur from flexion and reextension when the facets are anatomically asymmetrical or when there is faulty derotation.

posed weight for a reasonable period of time. If the object which a person must hold immediately before him is too heavy, muscular contraction may be insufficient. As the object is held farther away from the body, muscular tone decreases because the value of the fulcrum decreases. Holding even a reasonable weight at a reasonable distance from the body for too long a period of time will cause muscular fatigue or exhaustion.

Merely standing in a forward-flexed posture of 10 to 15 degrees causes excessive loading upon lumbar intervertebral discs. This forward-flexed posture can also be simulated in the seated forward-flexed position. These two positions are assumed in many occupations and are causative of industrial cases of low back pain.

When the muscular contraction needed to sustain this slightly flexed posture has been exhausted or overcome, the brunt of the stress falls upon the ligaments which have a limited resiliency and are capable of producing pain. In that flexed posture there is an increase of intradiscal pressure that can theoretically also cause pain.

61

The erector spinae muscles assuming a powerful isometric contraction eventually fatigue and by virtue of their fatigue and ischemia also become painful. Undoubtedly there is some periosteal irritation from persistent myofascial stress.

When muscular contraction has been overcome or exhausted the brunt of the stress falls on the ligaments which have a limited resiliency and once the ligaments give way the stress falls on the joints and subluxation of the joint results. Pain can manifest itself many times during this sequence of events. Sustained muscular contraction can produce ischemia in the muscle tissue, capable of causing pain. Excessive strain on the myofascial attachment to the periosteum may also result in pain. Painful capsular stretch may follow the loss of the ligamentous "protection" that normally guards the joints.

Any overwhelming stress will stretch the ligaments of the functional unit, exceed the movement within the unit and ultimately stretch the long ligaments throughout the entire spine. Not only segmental instability may result but it is possible that the physiologic curves of the spine may be altered. As previously stated, overwhelming stress may be caused by an extraordinary weight imposed on the supporting structure, by an average weight held in a markedly eccentric manner, or by a light object held for unduly long periods of time.

Normal Strain on Abnormal Back

Normal use of an abnormal back implies proper utilization of a structurally defective back. Sometimes due to a defect in the spine or its contiguous tissues, the stress may be improper or excessive. This defect may be found in the bony structures, the articular portions of the spine, the ligaments, the muscular tissues, or in any of these combinations.

In a *structural scoliosis* the facets are not parallel in a symmetrical plane because of the lateral curving and associated rotation of the vertebral segments. Bending and extending in an anterior posterior direction that occur normally at the lumbar segment must now be done with the facets in an oblique position. The gliding movement is attempted by the asymmetrical facets, and smooth movement of one pair of facets upon the other is impaired, with a loss of facile action and the limitation of total movement. When movement is forced past the point that the facet alignment will now permit, the joints will be driven together and impacted. This is rightfully called "impingement" or "freezing" of the facets.

Two different mechanics may cause pain in the movement of a scoliotic spine. Rotation of a segment of the spinal column decreases the range of normal physiologic movement of that segment. This limitation occurs because the facets now assume a position at an angle to their usual plane of action. The ligaments along the spine follow this curved line and thus shorten. Spinal flexion past a certain degree is met by mechanical structural restriction, and any exertion of force will result in overstretch of the tissues. In this type of movement restriction the pain mechanism initiated by forced flexion occurs from ligamentous-articular-capsular stretch.

The second pain mechanism attributed to scoliosis occurs as the spine reextends from the flexed position. As the spine extends and approaches the erect lumbar lordotic curve, the posterior articulations reapproximate. Parallel symmetrical facets with smooth synovial lining permit unimpeded reapproachment. The presence of facet asymmetry causes the female carriage to be oblique to the entering male portion of the facets, so that impingement can result.

If the patient violates the reverse of the lumbar pelvic rhythm in reassuming the erect posture (e.g., resumption of lumbar lordosis before there has been concomitant pelvic derotation and/or there has been inadequate derotation from the rotated flexed position), the facets can be "jammed" together (Fig. 47).

Disc degeneration resulting in functional instability can cause a "catch" on reassuming the erect posture. This is caused by excessive "shearing" of that specific functional unit when it is "out of sequence" with adjacent units during flexion and reextension (Fig. 48).

In many instances the *facet impingement* which has been termed "joint" dysfunction may persist and cause chronic pain and limitation. Careful examination reveals (1) tenderness over the involved functional unit, (2) limited movement of that segment in flexion or lateral flexion, and (3) tenderness over the specific zygapophyseal joint.

Normal use of an abnormal back resulting in pain occurs also when *tight hamstrings* are present. The lumbar spine is not abnormal, but the lumbar-pelvic rhythm has a malfunctioning cog in its mechanism. Full painless movement of the spine requires complete rotation of the pelvis as well as total reversal of the lumbar lordotic curve. Inflexible hamstring muscles by their attachment from the posterior knee region to the ischial tuberosity of the pelvis prevent full rotation. In total body flexion, once the pelvis has reached its maximum rotation, if total flexion has not been reached, further bending may be forced by more lumbar curving. As further bending of the lumbar spine is prevented by the posterior longitudinal ligaments, insistence will result in ligamentous stretch pain. Tearing of the ligamentous-periosteal fibrous attachment may actually result, if not a tear in the ligament itself. Repeated overstretching leads to instability of that segment, owing to the elongation of the restrictive ligaments (Fig. 49).

The "tight low back" produces pain in a manner converse to that of the tight restrictive hamstrings. In the tight low back mechanism the

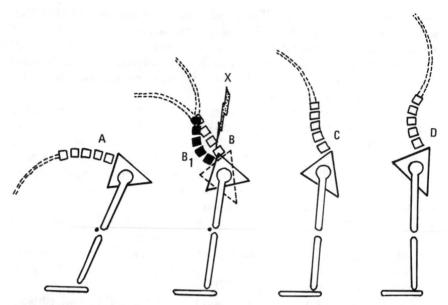

FIGURE 48. Mechanism of acute facet impingement. *A, B, C,* and *D* depict the proper physiologic resumption of the erect position from total flexion with reverse lumbar-pelvic rhythm. B_1 shows improper premature lordotic curve which cantilevers the lumbar spine anterior to the center of gravity. This position approximates the facets at X and, coupled with the eccentric leading of the spine, requires greater muscular contraction of the erector spinae group. Facet impingement can occur.

pelvic rotation phase of the lumbar-pelvic rhythm is free and full, but the lumbar-flexion phase is impeded. Instead of the lumbar lordosis physiologically flexing synchronously with the rotation of the pelvic area, the pelvis rotates and the lumbar curve, having gone as far as the tight paraspinous tissues will permit, ceases. At this point the low back attempts to flex further but cannot. Further forcing will cause painful stretching of the posterior longitudinal ligament and the fibrous elements of the paraspinous muscles.

Normal Stress on an Unprepared Normal Back

The third concept of body mechanics dysfunction that may result in low back pain is that of normal stress imposed on a normal back but imposed at a moment when the back is unprepared for such stress.

Any neuromusculoskeletal activity is preceded by anticipation and preparation. Muscular contraction, either isometric or isotonic, is needed to initiate movement. Under normal conditions an impending action will evoke appropriate action. The anticipated movement must be graded to the required intensity of contraction, to the rapidity of the

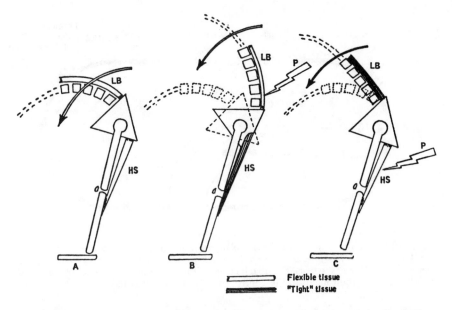

▭▭▭▭▭	Flexible tissue
▬▬▬▬▬	"Tight" tissue

FIGURE 49. Mechanism of stretch pain in the "tight hamstring" and the "tight low back" syndromes. A. Normal flexibility with unrestricted lumbar-pelvic rhythm. B. Tight hamstrings (HS) restricting pelvic rotation and thereby causing excessive stretch of low back (LB) resulting in pain (P). C. Tight low back (LB) performing an incomplete lumbar reversal and thus, by placing excessive stretch on the hamstrings (HS), causes pain (P) in both the hamstrings and the low back as well as a disrupted lumbar-pelvic rhythm.

contemplated action, and to the extent of contraction necessary for time and distance.

Contraction may "overshoot the mark" and cause excessive movement. Because this excessive movement exceeds the physiologic limitation imposed by ligaments, capsular and articular tissue damage occurs which may be micro- or macroscopic in degree but nevertheless results in pain and disability.

The movement must be considered not only as to the appropriate muscular effort, but also as to the exact direction of movement of the individual segments. The facets allow movement in a sagittal direction and prevent or restrict lateral movement. This is true in the erect or in the hyperextended position of the lumbar spine. As flexion occurs, the facets separate and allow increasingly more lateral and rotating movement (see Fig. 9).

In the flexed posture, rotation of the functional unit occurs to the extent of the facet; restriction then is limited only by the annular fibers and the long ligaments. Flexion and rotation movement exceeding physiologic limits is probably the greatest cause of annular fiber tearing of the intervertebral disc. The outer fibers having the greatest range of

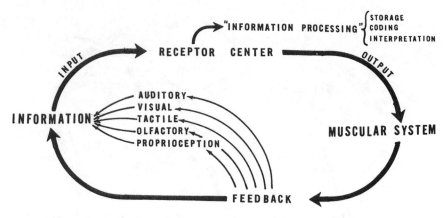

FIGURE 50. Information from internal and external environment via receptors. Process of learning a skill. Almost all behavior is motor in nature; man responds with voluntary and involuntary movements, which includes posture among others. Learning skills proceed in phases (see text). Feedback is one of the most important concepts in learning and is an important factor in the control of movement and behavior.

motion undoubtedly tear first and cause pain without signs and symptoms of frank herniation (see Chapter 5).

The term *normal* in relationship to movement requires discussion. Under average conditions *normal* muscular effort would be effective but not detrimental. As an example, lifting a suitcase considered empty would initiate appropriate muscular effort if the suitcase were empty, but be totally inadequate if the suitcase were heavily loaded. The resultant movement is obvious and can be stressful. The opposite is also predictable of what would result were the suitcase to be considered *heavy* and the muscular effort so graded only to result in excessive motion if the suitcase were empty.

Bending and reassuming the exact posture, lifting, and standing or sitting erect are all *learned activities.* These neuromuscular activities require good reflex activities of a genetic nature which have been coordinated, modified, and made more efficient by properly learned patterns of movement.

The central nervous system is influenced by numerous stimuli of which muscular activity affected by gravity is the major stimulus. Man modifies and controls his instinctive reaction, and muscular activity develops as a learned activity. These learned activities can be considered as skills (Fig. 50).

Learning skills proceed in three phases:

1. *Recognition of the plan* with its objective and goal. The efficacy of the information source must be determined. Sensory input has priorities since a man cannot contend with numerous stimuli

simultaneously. He selects one stimulus, most frequently a visual stimulus, and excludes or dampens the others. The attention span also influences how effective is the one source of information.

2. *Practice.* This is influenced by the complexity of the act, the desire or motivation to act, and the importance of the action. Feedback is important in the practice phase in determining frequency and intensity as well as correctness of the practiced act.

3. *Execution.* In this phase the neuromuscular system's output increases in ease and efficiency and decreases stress and anxiety. Actions become increasingly more automatic. If the action is proper, the proprioceptive phase is so coded. If the action is improper, an improper coding results and subsequent action, although incorrect, is interpreted as correct by the individual.

Just as they can be learned, skills can also be violated or misused by internal as well as external forces. A "tense," nervous person can act in an unusual, erratic manner. A fatigued person can move in an abnormal manner. An impatient person may violate a well-known learned pattern of bending or lifting. An angry person may do a movement that has been done properly for many years in an improper manner. All his previous skill momentarily is lost, and musculoskeletal injury results.

Electromyographic studies have confirmed the inefficiency of muscular effort in nervous, tense individuals. In the normal performance of a simple motor test requiring relatively few motor units, nervous or anxious people display simultaneous discharge of motor units throughout the entire body. Not only does this excessive motor activity cause inefficient energy expenditure, but also poorly integrated neuromuscular activity. A careful history usually elicits the mental status, the distracting situation, and the causative basis for faulty action that lead to musculoskeletal injury.

Each repeated condition that results in back pain undoubtedly leaves its residual damage to the tissues of the back until the degree of normalcy of the back decreases and a previously tolerable stress now becomes abnormal.

SUMMARY

Low back pain results from deviation of normal posture in the *static spine* and from deviation of normal function in the *kinetic spine*. Irritation of pain-sensitive tissues must occur before pain is elicited. Normal posture and normal kinetics in a normal spine do not initiate pain.

Low back discomfort in the *static* spine occurs primarily from an increase in the lumbosacral angle which in turn increases the lumbar lordosis. Most cases of postural low back pain must be attributed to an accentuated "sway back."

67

Low back pain resulting during or from movement of the spine can be attributed to violation of the *lumbar-pelvic rhythm*. The *rhythmic* pattern may be faulty in its performance or some of the functional segments of the spine that participate in the rhythm may be inadequate.

Any consideration of low back pain must keep in mind the factors of abnormal stress on the normal spine, abnormal stress on a mechanically normal spine, and the imposition of a usually normal stress on a mechanically normal spine but imposed at a time when the back is not ready to receive the stress.

It is now possible to turn to the patient who suffers from backache and apply to clinical use the knowledge of functional anatomy and the recognition of possible painful deviations.

BIBLIOGRAPHY

Altschule, M.D.: Emotion and skeletal muscle function. Med. Sci. 2(2):163-164, 1962.
Behan, R.C., and Hirschfeld, A.H.: The accident process II. Toward more rational treatment of industrial injuries. J.A.M.A. 186:300-306, 1963.
Hirschfeld, A.H., and Behan, R.C.: The accident process. J.A.M.A. 186:193-196, 1963.
Hirschfeld, A.H., and Behan, R.C.: The accident process III. Disability: acceptable and unacceptable. J.A.M.A. 197:2, 125-129, 1966.
Jacobson, E.: Electrical measurements of neuromuscular states during mental activities—Imagination of movement involving skeletal muscles. Am. J. Physiol. 91:567-605, 1930.
Jainsbury, P., and Gibson, J.G.: Symptoms of anxiety and tension and the accompanying physiological changes in the muscular system. J. Neurol. Neurosurg. Psychiatry 17:216-224, 1954.
Lundervold, A.: Electromyographic investigation during sedentary work—especially typewriting. Br. J. Phys. Med. 14:32-36, 1951.
Lundervold, A.: Electromyographic investigation of position and manner of working on typewriting. Acta Physiol. Scand. 24(Suppl. 84), 1951.
Weinstein, M.R.: The illness process. J.A.M.A. 204:3, 209-211, 1968.

CHAPTER 3

Clinical Application of Low Back Mechanics in the Diagnosis and Treatment of Pain Syndromes

The history and physical examination of the patient with low back pain must have as its objective a *functional* diagnosis based on static and kinetic appreciation of the patient's spine and its relation to the normal.

LOCALIZATION OF PAIN BY HISTORY-TAKING

It may be trite to say that the patient's claim of "pain in the low back" is not necessarily an accurate statement. Localizing the pain in the lower back region is the problem since the patient may be vague and obscure.

Many a patient will designate the wrong organ eliciting his pain, such as the patient with a pain in his "kidney area" when actually the pain exists in the lumbosacral area or the patient with a pain in his "hip" when the pain is really in the sacroiliac region. But the site of the pain can easily be localized if the patient is asked to point with his fingertips to the spot in pain. The site so specified has more anatomic localization than do the descriptive words of the patient.

A description of the characteristics of the pain is valuable. Words used by the patient, such as "dull," "sharp," or "burning," have significance in that certain tissues, when irritated, will cause pain of that specified type and description. The site of the tissues (responsible for this type of pain) in the functional unit or along the entire spine has obvious localizing value.

Frequency and duration of pain have both diagnostic and prognostic significance. Mechanical instability of the back can be suspected when

69

there is frequent recurrence of painful attacks. The duration of pain varies also with the type and site of tissue irritated. This gives insight into the recuperative powers of the patient. The amount of disability claimed by the patient to result from the pain gives the experienced examiner his first insight into the pain-threshold of the patient. The pain-tolerance of a patient is difficult to evaluate accurately.

After the localization of the pain has been determined, the case history will next seek the *"when"* and *"how"* of the pain-producing mechanism. A description of the *when* in relation to time of day or to type of work or activity is presented when the patient states, "It happens only when . . . ." The *when* thus also becomes a *how*, presenting some clarification of the mechanism of the pain production. The patient's description of the time and manner of the pain experience differentiates the pain in its *static* or *kinetic* nature.

PHYSICAL EXAMINATION

Examination is fundamentally an attempt to reproduce by deliberate actions and movements the patient's symptoms. A basic axiom follows: *If the characteristic pain can be produced by a position or by a movement, and the exact nature of that position and movement is completely understood, the mechanism of the pain production is understood.*

At precisely the position or the moment of the movement at which pain is produced, by knowing what is occurring in the body mechanics and by appreciating the deviation of this movement or position from normal function, the physician discovers the mechanism of pain production. As has been discussed, the history has already alluded to the general classification of static or kinetic, and the patient himself has suggested the *where, when,* and *how* of his pain. The examination now confirms the clinical impression implied by the history.

General Observations

The physical examination has already begun as the history is being taken. The manner in which the patient enters the office, and his sitting or standing posture as the history is recorded are significantly revealing. The static posture has already been observed, and an insight into the patient's emotional tone as portrayed by his postural attitude has been gained.

Likewise, the handshake, too often overlooked and too infrequently interpreted, is an exceedingly valuable portion of any physical examination. The basic personality often is revealed in a person's handshake.

70

The handshake is as revealing a depiction of the emotional tone as is posture.

The limp "dead fish" or "wet rag" handshake usually indicates a listless individual whose symptoms are in part influenced by this hypokinetic attitude and who can be expected to put very little effort into an energetic treatment program that the doctor will prescribe for him.

The "bone crushing" or "pump handle" handshake indicates a hyperkinetic, compulsive type in spite of the impression he wishes to create.

In contrast is the firm, reassuring handshake, when related to similar postural appearance and the objective history that is being noted, which gives the examiner a feeling of security in the integrity of the story the patient tells and confidence that the patient will try to carry out the prescribed treatment.

The history must carefully evaluate previous therapeutic attempts, and the reason for past failures must be judged carefully. Failure to improve from a program that once was deemed to be correct either stimulates a need for further studies or questions the accuracy of the patient's history. One or the other is in error.

The possibility of inaccurate diagnosis must also be considered. Again, failure of patient cooperation may indicate lack of understanding on the part of the patient or poor instructions that had been given by the former therapist. Another possibility must always be kept in mind, namely, that a patient may psychologically need his symptoms, either consciously or subconsciously, and will relinquish them reluctantly. This evaluation must be made very cautiously, but the truth may be suspected when the patient implies "happiness" over treatment failures, the knowledge that "everything has been tried" and that "the best doctors have been puzzled." The "pleasure from failure" is paradoxical but real.

The physical examination of the patient is best performed in a progressive-systematized pattern. This routine need not be stereotyped or inflexible, but the examination should be performed in an orderly sequence that tends to preclude omission of essential details.

The patient should be sufficiently undressed to permit adequate observation of the static and kinetic aspects of the body. The male patient can undress to his undershorts. The female patient must be exposed but must have protection against encroachment upon modesty. A gown of knee length which is open in the back but adequately fastened to permit movement should suffice for the examination.

The patient must be examined in the erect position, observed flexing forward, extending, in lateral flexion in both directions, and in rotation.

Every segment of the vertebral column must be evaluated and an attempt made to determine its contribution to pain as well as to limitation of movement.

The patient must be examined in the prone and in the supine positions. Tenderness must be elicited by palpating carefully and thoroughly pertinent portions of the back and lower extremities. Tissue changes such as tenderness and hyper- or hypoaesthesia must be sought. Segmental muscular "spasm" must be looked for by palpation. Both sides must be compared. A complete neurologic examination must be done, and a rectal examination completes the evaluation.

Evaluation of Posture (Static Spine)

The patient's posture has had a cursory examination when he enters the examining room and during the history portion of the interview. In the examining room the patient is intentionally and obviously examined for posture. He or she is aware of the scrutiny. This pose may be revealing. A pose may be assumed portraying what is considered to be proper posture, or it may be the pose that depicts the painful state or the feelings he wishes to portray. This projection of posture may be either unconscious or intentional, and the motivation is not always easily discerned. The posture assumed by the patient is always revealing, but the revelation assumes importance only insofar as it is correctly interpreted and properly used in diagnosis.

The examiner begins by observing the patient from a side view, with especial concentration on the lumbar curvature, the opposite curve of the dorsal spine, and the relative position of the hips, knees, and feet in relation to an assumed plumb line of gravity. The cervical spine, although not to be stressed here, cannot fail to be considered in the total aspect of body posture. This cervical curve must conform to the other curves and is a significant determinant of posture.

Pelvic Level—Leg Length

Posterior viewing of the static spine should first take into consideration the level of the pelvis. Determining the pelvic level is essentially an evaluation of leg length. To measure the length of each leg by tape measure from malleolus to anterior-superior spine or iliac crest is at best inaccurate and offers little practical significance. Ascertaining comparative leg lengths is of greatest value insofar as the legs through their upright supporting structure influence the level of the pelvis. This horizontal pelvic plane is the foundation of the spinal take-off, and its level can only be determined by examining the patient in the upright position.

72

The patient is examined standing barefooted with both legs close together and both legs fully extended at the knees. The pelvic level is then determined in three manners. The examiner places the fingertips of his hands upon the pelvic brim on each side. By sitting back, at arms' length, the examiner can determine the horizontal level of his fingertips and hence the level of the iliac crests. The accuracy of this measure is surprisingly precise and the differences of as little as one quarter of an inch can be estimated.

The "dimples" noted in most people in the region of the sacroiliac joints can be "lined up" by the eye and furnish another estimate of pelvic level. These dimples are located parasacrally where the gluteus maximus muscle attaches to the periosteum overlying the sacrum. Except in very obese or in very thin people, these dimples can easily be observed.

Observation of the lumbar spine in its take-off or in the angle of ascent from the sacrum presents a third method of determining pelvic level. The posterior-superior spines of the vertebrae are usually prominent and can be seen along the floor of the valley created by the erector-spinae muscle masses. The lumbar spine ordinarily takes off from the sacral base at right angles in a straight vertical direction. If an oblique take-off is noted, it indicates that the spine is curved or implies obliquity of the sacral base. These three methods of measuring leg length are used to determine the level of the pelvis only insofar as it influences lumbar spine take-off from its sacral base. The conclusion drawn from the three methods is significantly accurate.

If these three clinical methods of determining pelvic obliquity indicate any leg length discrepancy, the exact degree of leg length difference can be determined. Boards of known thickness can be placed under the foot of the short leg until the pelvis reaches the level determined by the above three methods. The thickness of the board establishes the degree of leg length difference. The boards of varying thicknesses of ⅛, ¼, ½, ¾, and 1 inch can be used in various combinations until the pelvic level has reached the horizontal. It must be remembered that a straight vertical spine, rather than a level pelvis, is desired. Achieving a level pelvis is merely a means toward this end.

When a significant leg length discrepancy exists, the cause of the difference will usually be revealed by further observations and appropriate studies. Unilateral *genu valgum* or *genu varum* may be a sufficient degree to cause a change in total leg length. Atrophy of a leg due to posterior poliomyelitis or to previous fracture or surgical intervention is easily discernible. Regardless of the cause, the significance of leg length shortening resides in its effect on the pelvic level and ultimately in its effect on the spinal alignment.

At this stage in the examination the static spine posture is evident.

The physiologic curves with their relationship to pelvic angulation have been ascertained, and the erectness of the spine from a posterior view has been sufficiently verified to assume proper facet alignment. The major factors influencing the static posture have been established so that it is possible now to consider the kinetics of the spine.

Lumbar-Pelvic Rhythm

Asking the patient to "bend forward in an attempt to touch your toes" but requesting that this flexion be done "without bending the knees" initiates the first phase of the lumbar-pelvic rhythm. These two requests have intentionally been placed within quotation marks. Observation of the bending forward "with knees stiff" permits evaluation of the freedom permitted rotation at the hip joints. Hamstring tightness is also revealed by this specific request. The stiff knees also insure maintenance of the horizontal pelvic level as ascertained from the posterior view of the static spine while leg length was being measured. A short leg that influences the static stance also must influence the kinetic spine by altering the vertical alignment of the spine. Bending one knee will cause that leg to be temporarily shorter than the fully extended leg.

"Bend *as if* to try to touch your toes" is requested of the patient because the ability to touch one's toes is not had by all and in no sense of the word implies normalcy. To infer that such flexibility is expected of the patient is fallacious insofar as a large percentage of people, regardless of their age, cannot, never have and probably never will be able to touch their toes, and yet are functionally adequate and flex in a pain-free manner. The main reason for asking the patient to perform this feat is to observe the *manner* of bending rather than to *measure* the *extent* of total flexion.

As the patient bends forward, the smoothness of the lumbar-curve reversal is observed. The ratio of this reversal is noted in respect to the pelvic rotation. The correlation of the two simultaneous movements is observed. In essence the lumbar-pelvic rhythm is studied. Each component of the movement is observed, and the relationship to each other in the rhythm is ascertained. Failure of the lumbar lordosis to reverse during flexion may indicate protective muscle spasm or mechanical restriction because of malfunction of the joints, capsules, ligaments, or muscles of the lumbar spine. Interruption of the pelvic rotation limiting the total lumbar-pelvic movement may imply tight hamstring muscles, irritable sciatic nerve, or inability of the pelvis to rotate on its hip-joint axis, owing to faulty hip joints.

The simultaneous lumbar-flexion action with the concomitant pelvic rotation should be a smooth action with each aspect being reasonably

74

complete. Restriction of either portion of the action indicates the phase of the rhythm that is defective.

If pain is elicited during the performance of this "bending forward" test, the observer must be immediately informed of the exact moment *when* the pain is felt and *where* it is felt. The "when" refers to the moment during the lumbar-pelvic flexion rotation at which the existence of pain is noticed and the "where" indicates the area of the back (or leg) at which the patient localizes the pain. Evaluation of the discrepancy in the rhythm, and the existence of pain at the moment when the discrepancy is noted reveals the mechanism of the pain. The "where" may denote a general area but when combined with a description of the pain intimates a more specific tissue site.

The patient himself indicates the "when" of the pain at the time the pain occurs during the bending exercise. This process fulfills the axiom "when I can reproduce pain and at the same time know what is happening, at that very moment I understand the mechanism of the pain."

Limited pelvic rotation around the transverse axis of the hip joints is frequently caused by "tight" hamstrings. Tight hamstrings signify inability of the muscles of the hamstring group to elongate because of excessive intramuscular connective tissue of limited elasticity. Usually the hamstrings which are inelastic bilaterally and symmetrically restrict pelvis rotation. Unilateral hamstring limitation will cause asymmetrical pelvic limitation in addition to a rotatory trunk flexion. Ultimate testing in straight leg raising range will reveal the extent of hamstring elasticity. Sciatic nerve-stretch pain also produces unilateral restriction of pelvic rotation and interferes with the smooth lumbar-pelvic rhythm.

The observation of the pathway traversed by the entire spine during its total flexion may reveal a functional scoliosis that in the static erect position was not apparent. Facet asymmetry may be revealed during flexion by its effect on the course and direction of the spinal flexion. Scoliosis may result, it must be remembered, by a pelvic obliquity caused by a short leg, and this scoliosis may become more apparent during spine flexion, even though it exists also in the erect posture.

Having observed the patient flex fully and slowly, and having observed the fulfillment of the flexion phase of the lumbar-pelvic rhythm, the physician will now ask the patient to return slowly to the erect position. After reaching the fully bent-over position, he must be warned that the reverse flexion be performed slowly.

Reversed lumbar-pelvic rhythm in extension is now to be observed. The gradual return of the lumbar flexion to the erect position of lordosis with smooth simultaneous reverse rotation of the pelvis to its physiologic sacral angle should be the exact reversal of the rhythm observed during flexion. During re-extension, the pelvis should grad-

75

ually resume its position over the plumb-line center of gravity. Proper "uncurling" should be smooth, symmetrical, and painless.

Should pain or discomfort be noted during re-extension, the exact moment and the exact point of the extension mechanism should be noted. At the instant in the re-extension cycle when pain is evoked, a discrepancy in the lumbar-pelvic rhythm can usually be observed. The most frequent divergence in the rhythm is that of a premature return of the lumbar spine lordosis with the reverse rotation of the pelvis lagging. The lumbar lordosis is resumed before the pelvis establishes itself beneath the lumbar curve and is adequately derotated. At this stage of re-extension the lumbar spine should be in its erect lordotic phase and the sacral base should have returned to its proper erect supporting angle, but we find the pelvis is still tilted and thus the take-off of the lumbar spine occurs in a forward slant. The lumbar spine is cantilevered anteriorly to the center of gravity.

Because of the premature lumbar lordosis, the spine is eccentrically loaded, and muscular action is needed to maintain it in this off-center balance. This position is inefficient and fatiguing. In its attempt to achieve balance over the proper center of gravity the lumbar spine will arc, that is, increase its lordosis and thus further approximate the posterior articulations. The combined "arching backward" and the added muscular contraction to maintain the eccentric balance further compress the facets together and cause them to become weight-bearing. Diagrammatically, the reverse of flexion is depicted in Figure 28, viewed in reverse, and the faulty mechanism of de-rotation is shown in Figure 51.

The kinetic examination proceeds with the patient continuing to arch further backward. This extension after the patient has reached his static posture is, therefore, a position of hyperextension. This maneuver further increases the lumbar lordosis, the posterior articulations are more approximated, the center of gravity moves backwards, and the pelvis must, therefore, shift forward to keep the patient in balance. A marked "sway back" is created by this position. If pain results, similar to that previously complained of by the patient, the mechanism of the pain is revealed. Increase of the lumbar lordosis with posterior articular approximation is the cause. It must be admitted that this extreme "arching backwards" cannot be considered a daily ritual or an everyday occurrence, but the mechanism of pain production is basic. The graphic "arching" due to hyperextension is depicted in Figure 49C, and the pelvic relationship to the center of gravity is clearly apparent.

So far in the examination the *static* or postural and *kinetic* or functional spine have been evaluated both from the lateral view and the anterior-posterior aspect. We may possibly have reduplicated the patient's pain and thereby have revealed the mechanism of pain produc-

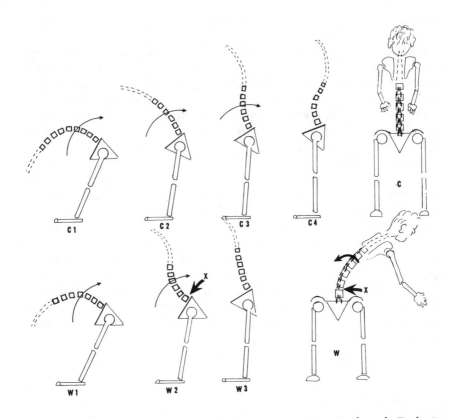

Figure 51. Faulty re-extension from the bent-over position. C_1 through C_4 depict gradual re-extension by simultaneously rotating the pelvis as the lumbar spine moves from reversed lordosis into erect lumbar lordosis. With the spine straight, as in C, the facets move properly. W_1 through W_3 depict improper re-extension where at W_3 the lumbar spine has become already "arched" before the pelvis has adequately rotated in a proper *lumbar-pelvic rhythm*. If the person is also rotated during this re-extension motion, his facets can "jam" during return to erect position, and the discs are subjected to additional stress from the torque motion.

tion. The severity of the pain may not have been reduplicated as the production of severe pain demands more factors than the circumstances of the examination permit. What is significant is the reproduction of the pain by a controlled position or action.

The lower extremities must also be considered. The hip-joint range of motion must be evaluated. Tenderness of the thigh and calf muscles as well as hyper- and hypoesthesia of the skin must be determined, atrophy noted, and circulation examined. All may implicate low-extremity pathology or findings referable to the lumbar spine.

The neurologic and skeletal examination will be discussed in greater detail in subsequent chapters, as will additional confirmatory tests.

SUMMARY

The patient who presents himself with a complaint of low back pain is evaluated by means of the case history and by specific physical examination. The history indicates *where, when,* and *how* the pain occurs. The *static* or the *kinetic* nature of the dysfunction is specified.

The *where* of the pain given in the history furnishes an anatomic localization; the *when* implies the time of movement, the nature of the movement, and the relationship to environmental factors that may be relevant. The *how* of the pain is divulged to the examiner who is cognizant of different mechanisms which may possibly cause pain. The characteristics of the pain described corroborates in part the suspected tissues involved as indicated in the history.

The examination, by permitting observation of *static* structure and the performance of *kinetic* function, leads to a functional diagnosis. If the normal is known regarding *static* and *kinetic* spinal function and appearance, the deviation from this normal can be appraised.

The axiom now applies: *If characteristic pain can be reproduced by a position or by a movement and the exact nature of that position and movement is fully comprehended, the mechanism of the pain is understood.*

CHAPTER 4

Comprehensive Therapeutic Approach to Low Back Pain

After a careful, complete evaluation by history of the causation of the low back pain, and verification of the mechanical basis of the pain, treatment is instituted. The objectives of treatment are:

1. alleviation of pain;
2. restoration of motion and mobility;
3. minimizing residual impairment;
4. prevention of recurrence;
5. intervention of entry into chronic pain.

ACUTE PAINFUL EPISODE OF LOW BACK PAIN

Frequently, an acute discomfort of the low back does not permit an immediate, thorough examination. Only a history may be elicited, and the patient presents limited flexibility, possible scoliosis, analgic spine, tenderness of the musculature of the lumbar area, and limited straight-leg raising.

Gross neurologic deficit can be ascertained with reasonable ease, but is usually not present in early lumbosacral pathology. Testing for a positive Laségue (SLR), gross sensory dermatome deficit, and gross motor loss of big toe extensor, anterior tibialis, quadriceps, and gastroc—all can be easily and rapidly discerned. The status of the lumbosacral plexus nerves that emerge from the lumbosacral spine are all evaluated by reflex examination and sensory dermatome mapping.

Pain can be modified by medication, rest, and modalities. *All must be utilized with positive reassurance and support from the examiner.* A brief explanation after a reasonably complete history and examination as to the cause, expected course, and projected treatment allays many fears that can enhance pain and disability. Words such as "spasm," "discogenic disease," "sciatica," and "arthritis" have no specific

79

meaning but may connote a frightening prospect to the patient.

Medications for relief of pain are best used on a specified basis of every 4 or 6 hours, depending on the duration (half-life) of the drug, rather than as requested by the patient. In patients prone to addiction or dependency drugs become a reward for pain and are difficult in later periods of illness to decrease or discontinue.

Most muscle "relaxants" are sedatives and are capable also of being depressants. They must be used carefully with these features in mind. Where bed rest is also contemplated, large initial doses are valuable. They must be given in limited doses and eliminated before they result in too much depression and discontinued when active participation in activities by the patient is required.

Oral anti-inflammatory medication is also valuable when given for a limited period of time, with careful explanation to the patient of possible side effects and with all the possible contraindications for the drug being considered. These drugs frequently permit lesser doses and duration of pain medication.

In patients who are or have been premorbidly depressed or who react to their acute impairment with depression, the early institution of antidepressant medication is valuable. Because most antidepressant psychotropic drugs do not become effective for three or more weeks, valuable time is gained.

Rest may be general or local. Generally, complete bed rest with elimination of gravity is beneficial. Bed rest demands a firm bed board under the mattress to prevent sagging in the middle. This requires a board at least ¾ to 1 inch thick. The mattress on such a board is used merely to contour the body to prevent pressure points on the bony prominences. A mattress 4 to 6 inches thick, sufficiently firm to buoy the body, is adequate. A water bed is well tolerated.

Bathroom privileges must be curtailed and controlled. In the case of male patients, bladder function can easily be controlled with a urinal or a wide-mouth bottle. Female patients may require some nursing assistance in the use of the bed pan. A bedside commode is best as it permits the patient to maintain the usual bowel-bladder function without frequent trips to and from the bed.

Medication given for pain often has a constipatory nature. This combined with pain and inactivity may encourage constipation with subsequent discomfort and "straining." Stool softeners or mild laxatives are of value. Proper toilet facilities are obviously the best assurance of good bowel habits.

The proper position in bed is the *position of comfort to the patient.* Some patients are comfortable in the fully extended supine position. Many, however, are most comfortable in the "semi-Fowler" position or the curled-up fetal position. In the mechanical hospital bed this posi-

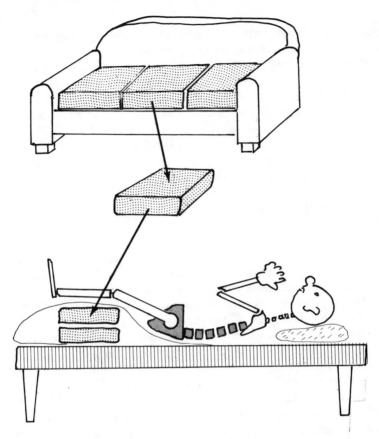

FIGURE 52. Home flexed bed posture utilizing square sofa pillows inserted under bedsheets to facilitate flexed hip and knee posture in lumbar discogenic disease.

tion can be easily achieved, but in the home it may present some problems.

To assume a semi-flexed position at home, placement of pillows under the knees is difficult to maintain and unreliable in determining the degree of flexion. One or more flat, square pillows, commonly found on most sofas, may be placed under the patient's knees. Placing these pillows *under* the bed sheets will allow them to remain more securely on the bed (Fig. 52).

In many cases of acute low back pain, 3 to 5 days of bed rest will suffice. Where there is severe antalgic spine limitation and scoliosis with radicular symptoms, 7 to 14 days are required. A minimum of 5 weeks has become routine in the treatment of the "acute disc hernia-tion."[1]

"*Rest*" is a term that can be interpreted in many ways. This interpre-tation must not be left to the discretion of the patient but must be clearly defined. How much of the day should one rest? How long is bed rest expected? For what purposes is getting out of bed permitted (bathroom privileges, meals, visitors, phone)?

Getting out of bed must be explained and even demonstrated:

1. Patient *must not* come to a straight sitting-up position in bed.
2. Patient must roll over on one side with hips and knees flexed and come up sideways.
3. Low back must be kept slightly flexed and immobile during entire movement.
4. Once feet are on the floor, patient must arise *slowly,* keeping body center of gravity over the feet, and *not extend* to full erect posture with full lumbar lordosis.

Whether or not to do bed exercises is also a subject of controversy. Some physicians advocate early gentle flexion exercises. Others avoid any movement and adhere to complete rest in the most comfortable position. These are individualized requirements.[2]

During the first few days most patients cannot or will not move with ease, and they should be allowed complete rest. By the third or fourth day, gentle flexion exercises will begin elongating the contracted muscles and promote the gradual recovery of patients who do not have significant subjective and objective signs of radiculitis. These exercises can be initiated with simultaneous use of a modality.[3]

Numerous modalities have been advocated. During the early acute painful state with much protective spasm (antalgic spine and/or functional scoliosis), local ice application has definite merit.[4-6] Local application of ice over a muscle probably acts on the muscle's spindle system. A muscle that retains its extensibility to its normal resting length is usually pain-free. When it does not retain its extensibility, it is considered to be in "spasm" and a source of pain.

Ice applied to the overlying skin is considered to send impulses to the cord that compete with the pain-producing impulses that are conveyed by much slower fibers. The ice-produced impulses temporarily cause a refractory period in the other impulses, and muscle spasm is momentarily relieved. Stretch of the muscle is now possible, which decreases the spasm.[7]

If ice is applied for too long a period, the muscle may be chilled, which increases the spasm. Application, therefore, must be in a definite stroking direction along the muscle fibers. Ice can be applied by use of ice cubes, ethyl chloride spray,* or Fluorimethane† spray. A specific technique of spraying has been advocated by Travel.[8]

---

*Ethylchloride is potentially explosive and flammable.

†Fluorimethane spray is manufactured by Gebauer Chemical Company, Cleveland, Ohio.

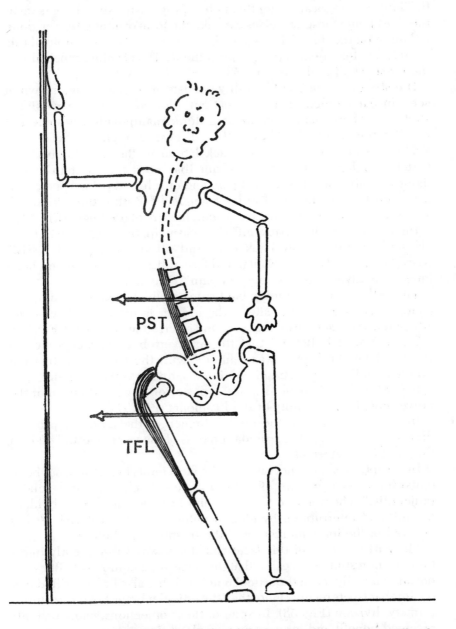

FIGURE 53. Lateral trunk flexibility exercises. By leaning sideways against a wall with both feet sufficiently far from the wall to shift the center of gravity, the spine will bend laterally toward the wall. The paraspinous tissues (PST) toward the wall on the convex spinal side will be stretched. The tensor fascia lata (TFL) on that side nearest the wall will also be stretched during this exercise.

After spraying the patient's low back where the light painful "spastic" muscles are located, gentle gradual progressive stretching is instituted. At home these exercises can take the form of gentle flexion done in bed or on the floor. The "knee chest" exercise is an example of this exercise. Lateral flexion done against the wall[9] is of value, especially in the presence of scoliosis (Fig. 53).

If restriction of lateral flexibility persists or scoliosis remains when seen in early office visits, the patient's low back can be passively stretched. These maneuvers are considered manipulation by some and mobilization by others. They will be discussed in greater detail.[10,11]

There is an area of the low back lateral to the fifth lumbar (L_5) vertebra and medial to the posterior iliac crest that contains many tissues capable of causing local pain and/or referred pain. This region has been termed the "multifidus triangle,"[12] Within this "triangle" are located many tissues that have been the site of treatment (Fig. 54).

Interruption of low back muscle spasm in this region has been claimed to relieve low back pain and eliminate a positive SLR (Laségue) test.[13] Local muscular and fascial tissues in this region have long been advocated as sources of pain[14] (Fig. 55).

This is the area of the iliolumbar ligament which has been claimed as a site of pain[15] and in the site of the lumbar facets which have been attributed as the source of local pain and referred sciatic pain[16] (Fig. 56).

The claim of Kellgren[17] that the intervertebral ligaments were a source of low back pain was refuted[18] with the conclusion that the original studies of injecting hypertonic saline into the ligaments had actually involved injections into the posterior primary division of the nerve roots in the vicinity of the ligaments (Fig. 57).

In the lumbar region the medial branch of the posterior primary division runs close to the articular process of the vertebrae and ends in the multifidus muscles.

Interruption of the innervation of the facet joints in this area has been considered as a means of relieving low back pain and sciatic radiculitis.[19] The nerve to the facet joint has been anatomically identified,[20] and interruption by electrocautery under direct vision[21] has evolved in the implementation of the treatment technique.

The early success of this facet rhizotomy was subsequently questioned when studies revealed that the invasion techniques of Rees did not anatomically reach the articular nerve. It has also been verified that the lumbar facets receive more than the articular branch of the posterior primary division (Fig. 58). In spite of these objections, many patients received benefit and for varying periods of time.

Changes of the functional unit that result when there is disc degeneration or rupture that permit axial forces to place stress on the contiguous tissue such as the facet joint, the annulus, the ligaments, or the

84

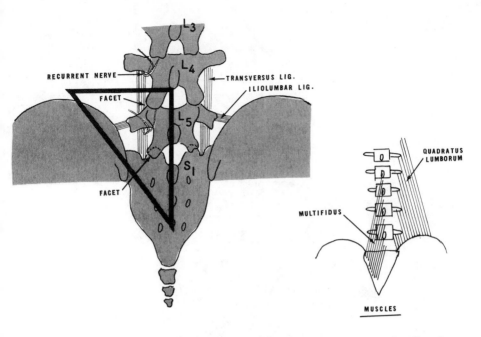

FIGURE 54. Multifidus triangle. This is an arbitrary triangular area extending from L_4 to the iliac crest and down to the sacrum, containing numerous pain-producing tissues, including facets, facet innervation, transversus ligament, quadratus lumborum muscle, multifidus muscle, iliolumbar ligament, and fascia.

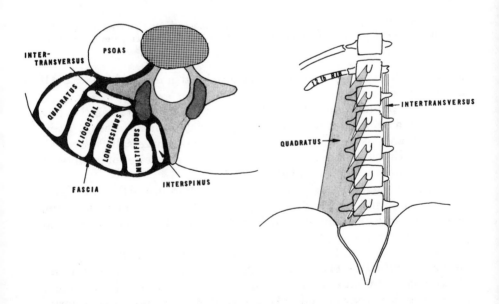

FIGURE 55. Muscles and fascia within the multifidus triangle.

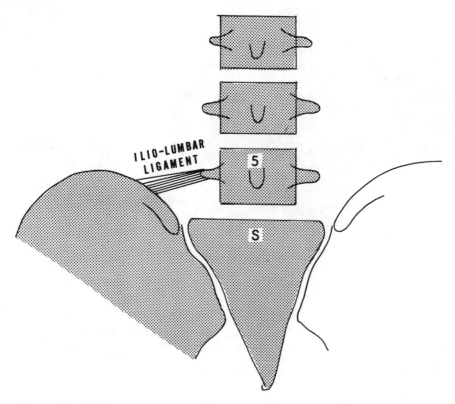

FIGURE 56. Iliolumbar ligament. This ligament connects the transverse process of the fifth lumbar vertebra to the iliac crest. Its function is that of stabilizing the L_5 vertebra.

muscles of the vertebral column can cause local or referred pain.[22-24] All of these tissues are found in the "triangle."

"Trigger points" of myofascial tissues have long been related to low back pain as either local sites or points of sclerotomal referral. Their histopathology is neither fully understood nor universally accepted, yet their clinical presence has been verified, and relief of symptoms from treatment is commonplace.

Of these "trigger points" the quadratus lumborum and the multifidus muscle are implicated as sites and sources of localized low back pain. Recently, more distal myofascial "trigger points" have been correlated to acupuncture points.[25]

Sites of referral to the posterior iliac crest area from $T_{12}L_1$ thoracolumbar vertebral units are also located near the "triangle," but reproduction occurs from vertebral column manuevers at the T_{12}-L_1 area.[26] Usually in this syndrome lateral movement of the T_{12} posterior superior spine or direct pressure upon that process elicits tenderness. There is

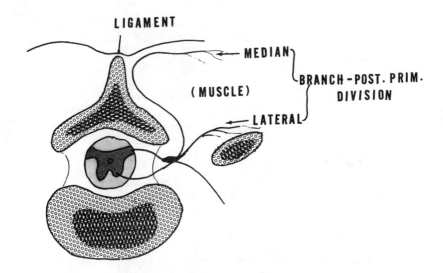

LIGAMENT

←— MEDIAN⌉
(MUSCLE) ⌊BRANCH–POST. PRIM.
DIVISION
←— LATERAL⌋

FIGURE 57. Posterior primary division. This demonstrates no innervation to the posterior spinous ligament which is known to be sensitive.

also deep tenderness in deep friction pressure upon the unilateral facets at that level (Fig. 59).

The referral site at the iliac crest reveals deep, specifically localized tenderness (digital) at the edge of the ilium, and there is sensitivity of the skin in that region during the process of "skin-rolling." Muscular modules that are firm and tender may be felt in that iliac crest region (Fig. 60).

Confirmation of this particular painful site with its origin at the thoracolumbar vertebral segment is done by injecting 1 to 2 ml of anesthetic agent 2 cm lateral to the posterior superior spinous process into the facet area. Rotatory manipulation of the thoracolumbar region is also therapeutic, as is a local injection lateral to the thoracolumbar junction.

The lumbar spine, by virtue of its facets, moves in flexion-extension. The thoracic spine moves in lateral flexion, by virtue of the plane of the facets but not in flexion-extension. The only site where rotation can occur is at the transitional vertebral segment, the thoracolumbar junction (T_{12}-L_1).

Rotation at this transitional level is limited by its facets. Excessive movement here can cause root entrapment with referral of pain down the posterior primary division to the region of the iliac crest. Rotatory manipulation performed by rotating the thoracic spine upon the fixed pelvis can restore mobility of the juncture (Fig. 61).

Manipulation of the lumbar spine, usually performed by rotation of the lumbar segment with the spine flexed and the pelvis fixed, will

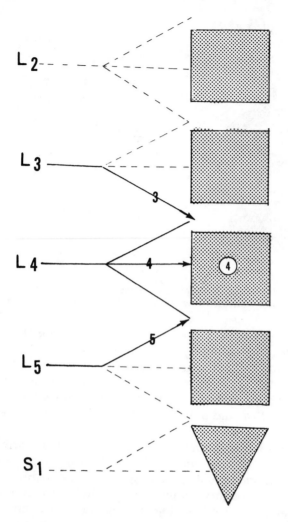

FIGURE 58. Multiple innervation of facets. Each facet receives its specific branch of the posterior primary division and a branch from the nerve roots cranial and caudal to it.

restore lumbar flexibility and disengage the facets, thus relieving the "entrapped" nerve root (Fig. 62). This manuever is performed by also pulling distally upon the iliac crest which laterally flexes the lumbar spine with simultaneous rotation.

The concept of Maigne "manipulation in the direction of no pain," and therefore of less resistance, is effective.[27] With painful or limited movement to the left, the therapeutic manuever is to the right.

Manipulation must *not* be violent or forceful. Full passive range of motion is gained with full relaxation of the patient, though a brief thrust

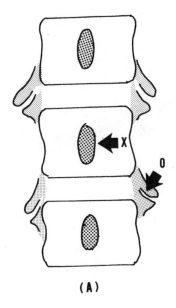

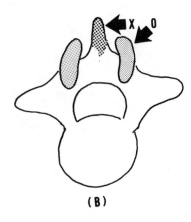

(A)

(B)

FIGURE 59. Tender spots over vertebral sites of pathology. A. Lateral pressure at the posterior-superior spine (X) elicits pain at the affected segment. B. Deep tenderness can be elicited by pressure over facet joints (O).

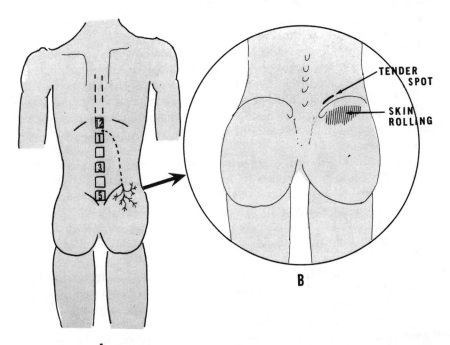

A

B

FIGURE 60. Referred pain from thoracolumbar articulation. Pain can be referred to the posterior-superior iliac crest via the posterior primary division of the T_{12} nerve. Insert shows the site of tenderness near the region of hyperesthetic skin from the T_{12}-L_1 radiculitis.

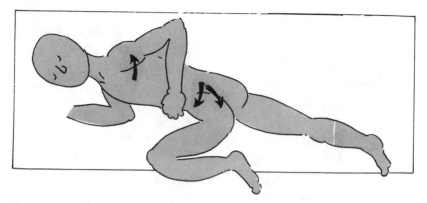

FIGURE 61. Manipulation of the thoracolumbar junction. With the patient positioned on the treatment table, the superior leg is flexed, the lower leg extended, and the lumbar spine flexed. With counter ("fixing") pressure against the superior shoulder, the upper trunk is maximally rotated. The lower movement is exerted against the iliac crest downward and in the opposite rotation to the upper force. When range is reached passively, a small "thrust" further dislodges the vertebrae.

in that direction through a short distance is the usual manipulation thrust (Fig. 63). An audible "crack" or "snap" is not mandatory to signify a successful manipulation.

The thrust must be precise, controlled, in the right direction, and at the specific vertebral segment. The thrust must be imparted to the patient only when the full passive range has been reached or the result will be inefficient. The patient must be fully relaxed, which means careful positioning, gentle handling, and reassurance, achieving a comfortable position for the patient and a careful, efficient position for the manipulator.

Experts in manipulation tend to oppose early manipulation of the patient with acute low back pain in which the patient exhibits the antalgic posture, functional scoliosis, and subjective radicular pain, and *do not* recommend manipulation until after a period of bed rest and relaxation. Others feel that early manipulation initiates immediate relief and faster recovery. This decision depends upon the experience of the physician.

Traction has gained the reputation of being "specific" treatment for the herniated lumbar disc. Traction in the manner and force usually applied *does not* distract the vertebrae but decreases the lordosis, thus separating the facets and opening the foraminae. It also gradually overcomes the spasm of the erector spinae muscles. By horizontal application to the patient, traction eliminates gravity (Fig. 64).

Pelvic traction is the most physiologic, the most comfortable, and the easiest to apply and to maintain. A snug pelvic band from which the traction is exerted fits above and on the iliac crest of the pelvis. Lateral

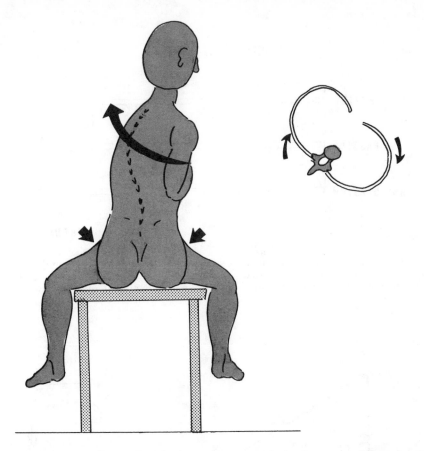

FIGURE 62. Rotatory manipulation technique. With the patient straddling the treatment table, the pelvis is "fixed." The upper trunk is rotated slowly to maximum by manual pressure on the left posterior rib cage and traction on the right arm-shoulder. The thoracic spine is rotated as shown in the drawing at right. Upon reaching maximum range, a gentle but firm thrust disengages the "locked" vertebral segment.

bands attached to the pelvic band (Fig. 65) exert equal pull on the left and right side, and must be placed posteriorly to "lift" the pelvis, which thus decreases the lordosis. The lateral bands are separated by a spreader bar.

The standard pelvic belt traction does not take into consideration the friction of the body weight to the bed or the treatment table. This site of friction creates a fulcrum point about which the pelvis rotates and conceivably increases the lordosis (Fig. 66). A single-strap pelvic traction belt has been designed which minimizes this mechanical disadvantage.

Recent medical literature has advocated total body weight traction applied in the hospital environment in a mechanical circular bed[28] (Fig. 67). This utilizes the concept that 30 percent of the total body weight is

RANGE OF MOTION

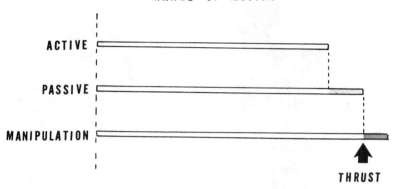

FIGURE 63. Concept of manipulation. A joint has an active range of motion that can passively be physiologically exceeded. When that range is reached, a firm but gentle thrust achieves the desired "joint play" that restores motion that frequently is lost.

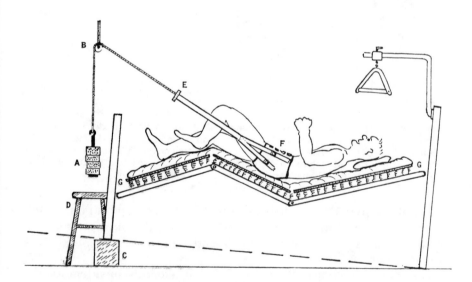

FIGURE 64. Pelvic traction with the patient in a "semi-Fowler position." The patient is wearing a pelvic band with the pull acting so as to flex the lumbar spine.
A. Weights applying the traction, usually 20 lbs.
B. Overhead pulley so placed that the pull tilts or lifts the pelvis.
C. Ten-inch block to elevate foot of bed.
D. Stool to support the weights when patient temporarily disengages them.
E. Spreader bar to separate the lateral straps pulling on the pelvic band around patient's pelvis.
F. Pelvic band with buckles to permit easy detachment by patient.
G. Split board between mattress and box springs to prevent sagging.

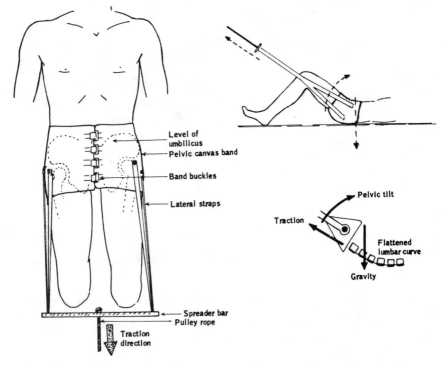

Level of umbilicus
Pelvic canvas band
Band buckles
Lateral straps
Spreader bar
Pulley rope
Traction direction

Pelvic tilt
Traction
Flattened lumbar curve
Gravity

FIGURE 65. Equipment for pelvic traction. Drawing at left depicts methods method of attaching pelvic traction equipment. The lateral straps are placed to permit leg movements and exercises in bed. Drawing at right discloses the resultant pelvic rotation gained by this method of applying traction.

found below the third lumbar vertebra.[29] If the patient is suspended at the thoracic cage, this amount of weight is applied as lumbar traction.

The traction belt is a harness that is comfortably fitted to the rib cage with the lowest strap *under* (below) the lowest ribs (Fig. 68).

Initially the bed is tilted to approximately 30 degrees of incline and gradually increased to 90 degrees (full erect posture), applying maximum traction of the lower body weight. Traction of 4 hours' duration is usually well tolerated, and as the increased vertical angle is gained, duration of traction is also increased (Fig. 69).

The harness is removed periodically during the day for skin care and to rest the patient. During this rest period the patient assumes complete recumbency with no standing, sitting, or walking except for bathroom privileges.

While in traction a foot plate is adjusted to be placed several inches below the patient's feet. This allows full traction and prevents the patient from sliding off the mattress in the event that the traction belt

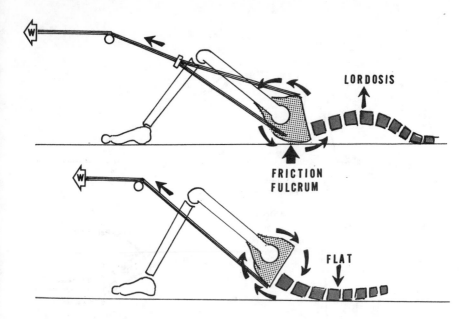

FIGURE 66. Pelvic traction principles. In the upper drawing the friction of the bed with the buttocks acts as a fulcrum about which the pelvis rotates to increase the lordosis. In the lower drawing the strap under the pelvis pulls to elevate the pelvis and decrease the lordosis.

becomes loosened. Traction is applied during waking hours for a period of 1 to 4 weeks. Leg exercises are encouraged during traction, as is pelvic tilting. Home traction making use of this principle is possible by means of a plywood tiltboard which is commercially available.

In the hospital setting this traction is applied within the electrically operated Stryker bed which controls the degree and duration of the angle of traction.

INJECTIONS

At the end of a reasonable period of complete bed rest and pelvic traction, with all modalities and medications *properly conducted,* a variation in treatment can be considered if symptoms persist. The "reasonable" period is usually considered to be approximately 10 to 14 days.

Before meaningful treatment of sciatic type pain can be initiated it is incumbent upon the physician to determine the exact site of nerve irritation[30] (Fig. 70).

Pain from disc herniation and compression of a *nerve root* can be reasonably concise: root distribution of pain, hyperalgesia, hypasthesia, motor root paresis and a positive straight leg raising. Pain

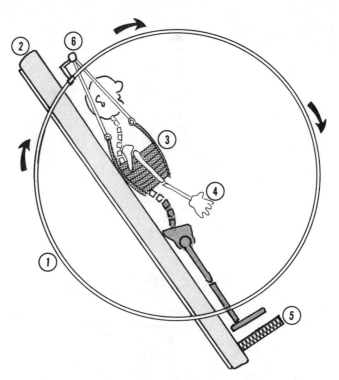

FIGURE 67. Gravity lumbar traction: (1) lumbar traction applied in a hospital setting with a circular bed; (2) mattress with bedboard within Stryker Circ-O-Lectric bed; (3) chest harness with lower straps under the rib cage and upper straps firmly grasping the rib cage; (4) bed manually controlled by patient; (5) footplate several inches below patient's feet for security; (6) snap ring attached to bed frame.

usually radiates below the knee. There is also an antalgic spine with scoliosis.

When the pain arises from the posterior primary division or from the recurrent sinuvertebral nerve distal to the foramen the precise site of nerve irritation can influence the treatment and its expected benefit. This latter type of pain has been termed pseudoradicular.[31]

In the pain originating from the posterior primary division (from muscles, ligaments, or the facets) there usually is no neurologic deficit, and there may be a minimal or equivocal straight leg raising test. Diagnostically, and therapeutically, an anesthetic injection of the posterior primary division nerve (L_{3-4-5}) at the level of the intertransversus ligament will relieve the pain. If this occurs and the pain has tended to become resistant to treatment, electrocautery of the posterior primary ramus can be performed with gratifying results.

Pain occurring from irritation of the recurrent sinuvertebral nerve will not be relieved by an anesthetic injection of the posterior primary nerve. This pain is mediated from irritation of the posterior longitudi-

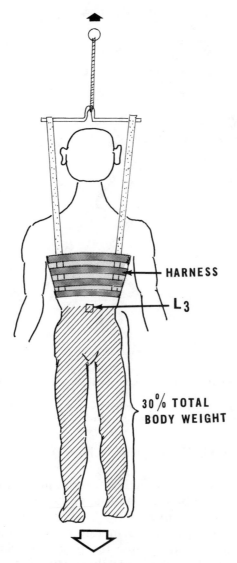

HARNESS

L₃

30% TOTAL BODY WEIGHT

FIGURE 68. Gravity lumbar traction. Based on 30 percent of total body weight below the third lumbar (L₃) level, traction is applied by supporting the body from a chest harness.

nal ligament, the anterior dura, of the apophyseal joints. The findings here also are merely a suggestive straight leg raising test with a *negative neurologic* examination and pain *not* radiating below the knee.

These patients can benefit from epidural injection of steroid and an anesthetic agent (30 cc of 0.5 percent procaine and 80 mg depromedral). Use of intradural steroids with an anesthetic agent has no effect upon

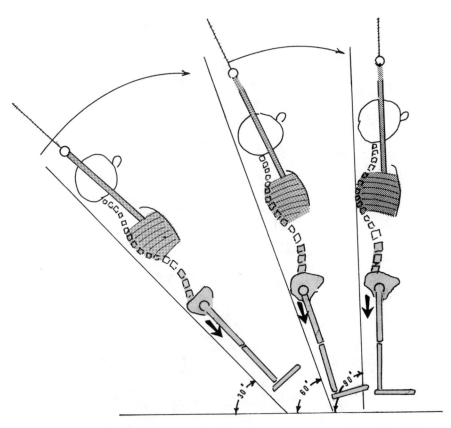

FIGURE 69. Gravity lumbar traction. As the bed (traction) angle is increased from 30 degrees to 90 degrees full upright, the amount of traction increases. The duration of traction can be determined.

the recurrent sinuvertebral nerve[32] and is effective only if there is inflammation of the root and its dural sheath (as in HNP and arachnoiditis).

It is conceivable that both posterior primary nerve root injection and epidural steroid-anesthetic injection should be undertaken before further diagnostic and therapeutic attempts are made.

Steroids have been considered effective in decreasing dural and nerve inflammation. Steroids can be given orally or intramuscularly as well as locally. Orally or intramuscularly an effective dosage sequence has been a large initial dose of 80 mg the first day, followed by 60 mg the second, 48 mg the third, then 36, 24, 18, and 12 mg, terminated at the end of 7 days. The sequence originally recommended in the literature was 64, 32, 24, 12, 8, 8, 8 mg of dexamethasone.[33] All the precautions of administering steroids must be observed (e.g., divided doses, use with

97

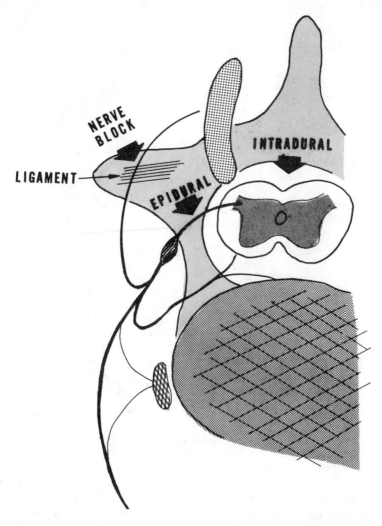

FIGURE 70. Differential diagnosis of site of radicular pain. By getting relief of "sciatic-like" pain from a nerve blocking the posterior primary division at the level of the intertransversus ligament, the site of pain is thus specified as being an irritation of that root. Relief from epidural steroids implicates inflammation of the sinuvertebral nerve. Benefit from intradural steroids indicates nerve root and dural inflammation.

meals, provision of antacids, and avoidance in patients with hypertension or diabetes).

Steroids have been advocated by the intradural and the epidural route. The intradural route requires using steroids that will be pharmacologically accepted intradurally and these are limited. All the precautions and contraindications of lumbar puncture are to be observed.

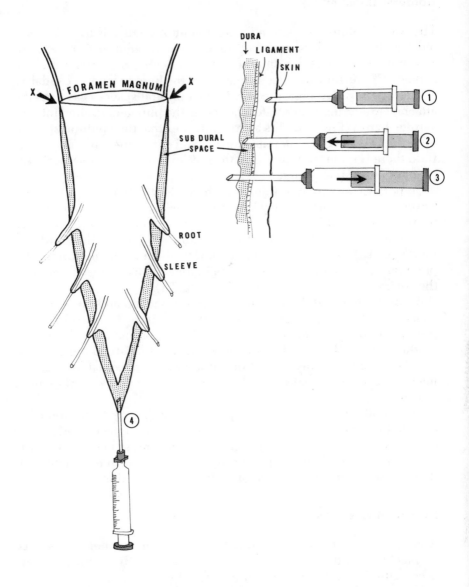

FIGURE 71. Dural sac with closure at the foramen magnum and the nerve root sleeves following the nerve roots through the intervertebral foramen. 1. Penetration of skin with spinal needle. 2. Penetration of ligament into subdural space with the vacuum pulling the plunger into the syringe. 3. Penetration of dura into spinal canal with the spinal fluid ejecting the plunger from the syringe. The steps are the signs utilized by the physician performing an epidural or intradural injection to determine the depth before injection. 4. Site of needle entrance into epidural sac for caudal injection.

Epidural Injection

The use of epidural injection for treatment of sciatica is over 40 years old.[34] Either steroids or anesthetic agents can be administered epidurally with benefit and minimal risk when all precautions are observed.[35,36] The route of injection can be at the lumbar level or caudally.

There is negative pressure within the epidural space, so as a needle attached to a syringe penetrates the space, the plunger is pulled into the syringe barrel (Fig. 71). This action indicates that the epidural space is entered if the needle penetrates further and enters the dura. The spinal fluid there is under pressure, and the outflowing spinal fluid forces the plunger out of the syringe.

To perform an epidural injection, the patient is seated in a forward-flexed position with his back to the physician. A 17-gauge Touhy thin-walled needle with a Huber point is recommended. The space between the second and third lumbar disc (L_2-L_3), or the third and fourth (L_3-L_4), is located. The injection is given in the midline. After penetrating the skin to a depth of approximately 3 cm, resistance from the interspinous ligament is met (see Fig. 71).

At this point the stylette of the needle is removed and the syringe is attached with the plunger inserted halfway into the barrel. As the plunger is drawn into the barrel (indicating a vacuum effect), the epidural space is entered. Air is now injected to distend the epidural sac. At this point a vinyl or Teflon catheter can be passed through the needle into the epidural sac, and the intended injection material can be injected.

Ten to 30 ml of solution, constituting a 0.25 percent solution of an anesthetic agent with or without steroid, is now injected. After one quarter of the solution is injected, aspiration must be performed to ascertain that no blood or spinal fluid has returned. Injection must be done slowly and steadily to avoid any vascular motion.

Intradural Injection

A lumbar puncture once performed in the routine manner can be used to inject steroid directly into the spinal canal. Specific steroids that are acceptable to the intradural route should be used.

Differential spinal anesthetic blocks have been advocated to determine which specific nerve fibers are involved. Originally this test was used to decide between "organic" pain and psychological pain, but the advocates of this purpose are fewer.

To perform a differential spinal block test, the patient must be cooperative, alert, and sufficiently intelligent to understand and cooperate. Before performing the test the patient must be tested carefully for pin-prick and light test appreciation and for area-mapping. Skin temperature must be tested and rated. All muscles of the specific nerve levels must be tested and graded.

The intradural injection site for the test is best performed at the specific level clinically established as the site and level of the pathology. This is usually the level of the L_4-L_5, L_5, and occasionally L_3-L_4.

Initially, 5 ml of normal sterile saline is injected. If the patient experiences marked or significant relief of pain from this injection, a large psychogenic factor is considered, and further testing may be discontinued.

With the needle left in place, the next injection is 5 ml of 0.2 percent procaine in isotonic saline. This blocks sympathetic nerves, thus relief being felt from this dilution of injected material indicates that treatment mediated through the sympathetic system may be of value. A lumbar paravertebral sympathetic block here may then be considered.[37,38]

A third injection is then administered of 5 ml of 0.5 percent procaine. This solution strength blocks the sensory fibers of the nerve roots. This test verifies nerve root pain, and failure to afford relief to the patient again indicates strong psychological factors.

Nerve Root Blocks

Nerve roots can be selectively infiltrated to specifically identify the exact nerve root or roots involved in the radiculites. This is a difficult test technically and requires an x-ray image intensifier to locate and identify the specific anatomic region.

The patient is placed in the prone position and a hemostat or another metallic object is taped upon the patient's back to localize the surface skin area after the x-ray is taken. A screen may be constructed for this purpose (Fig. 72). Such a screen also localizes the exact site of the facet joints.

The fifth lumbar root (L_5) is infiltrated by inserting an 18-gauge spinal needle at a 45-degree angle to the sagittal plane 6 cm lateral to the midline and 4 cm cephalad to the transverse process of the fifth lumbar root as located under fluoroscopy. The first sacral nerve (S_1) root is reached by injection into the sacral foramen (Fig. 73).

Facet Injection

The facet injection site has been discussed in this chapter in the section on the multifidus triangle (see Fig. 54). Hirsch[39] injected hypertonic saline solution into a facet joint and caused back and thigh pain. Injection into the third and fourth lumbar (L_3-L_4) facet produced pain down

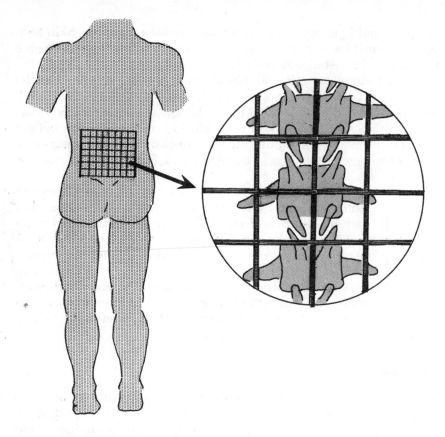

FIGURE 72.   Grid localizer for interarticular (facet) injection. A wire grid is placed upon the back of the prone patient and then x-rayed. The exact wire intersection overlying the facet can be localized on the patient. Injection can be made without an image intensifier, thus decreasing patient exposure to irradiation.

the anterior aspect of the leg, and the fifth lumbar-first sacral disc radiates the pain toward the ischium and buttocks.

Facet injections are best performed under fluoroscopic vision. With the patient laying prone, the same metal marker (or screen) as used in doing nerve blocks localizes the facet (see Fig. 72). A 3½-inch long 18- or 20-gauge needle is inserted approximately 1 inch lateral to the midline and directed straight down until bone is contacted. The superior facet is contacted and identified under fluoroscopy. Gentle movement caudally or cephalad of the needle tip can then place the needle into the joint. A "popping" sensation or sound is often experienced by the patient or the operator when the joint is entered. Some discomfort is experienced until the local anesthetic takes effect. Injection of 3 to 4 ml Conray 60 solution may be used to perform an orthogram, indicating

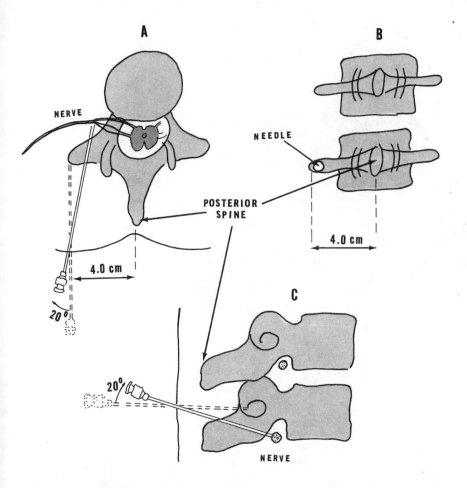

FIGURE 73. Technique for nerve root injection. With the patient in the prone position and with a pillow under the belly, the needle (8-10 cm, 21-gauge) is inserted 4 cm lateral to the *upper* margin of the spinous process until it penetrates to the lower margin of the transverse process (*B*). Upon contact the needle is withdrawn and inserted medially (*A*) and downward (*C*) about 20 degrees. Passing inferiorly to the transverse process (*C*), the needle is inserted until the nerve root is contacted, and the patient feels sudden sharp pain in the distribution of the root dermatome.

that the joint has been entered. Either an anesthetic or steroid or both is then injected.

All of the treatment modalities and techniques discussed above are attempts to interrupt the pain cycle depicted in Figure 74 via the posterior primary division and its branches or tissues supplied; the nerve roots at the intervertebral foramen or within, extradurally or intradurally; or at the anterior primary division.

103

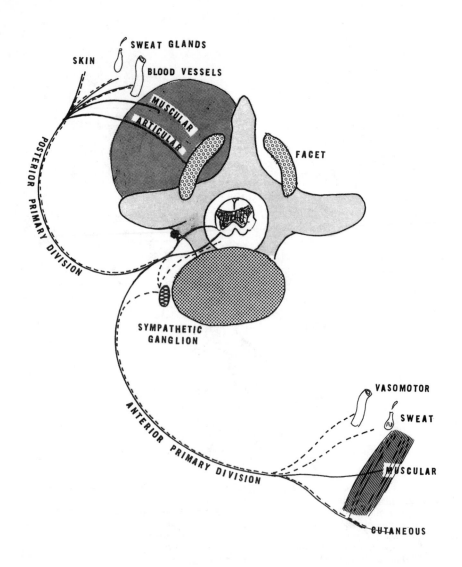

FIGURE 74. Neurologic pain pathways. A simplistic neurologic pathway is depicted, via anterior and posterior primary rami through which pain sensation is mediated.

This progression of treatment is undertaken to restore proper posture, proper muscle tone, adequate flexibility, proper psychological attitude, and proper body mechanics. In essence it was faulty mechanics that led to the appearance of low back pain and could cause a recurrence.

104

REFERENCES

1. Bed rest and lumbar disc protrusions. Br. J. Med., July 15, 1967, pp. 127-135.
2. Pearce, J., and Moll, J.M.H.: Conservative treatment and natural history of acute lumbar disc lesions. J. Neurol. Neurosurg. Psychiatry 30:13, 1967.
3. Lidstrom, A., and Zachrisson, M.: Physical therapy on low back pain and sciatica. Scand. J. Rehab. 2:37-42, 1970.
4. Newton, M.J., and Ruhl, D.: Muscle spindle response of body cooling, heating and localized muscle coolant. J. Am. Phys. Ther. Assoc. 4(2):91-105, 1965.
5. Mennell, J.M.: The therapeutic use of cold. J. Am. Osteopath. Assoc. 74:1146-1158, 1975.
6. Grant, A.E.: Massage with ice (cryokinetics) in the treatment of painful conditions of the musculoskeletal system. Arch. Phys. Med. Rehab. 45:233-238, 1964.
7. Mathews, B.H.C.: Nerve endings in mammalian muscle. J. Physiol. (Lond.) 78:1-53, 1933.
8. Travel, J.: Ethyl chloride spray for painful muscle spasm. Arch. Phys. Med. Rehab. 33:291-298, 1952.
9. Cailliet, R.: Low Back Pain Syndrome. ed. 2. F.A. Davis, Philadelphia, 1977, p. 76.
10. Bourdillon, J.F.: Spinal Manipulation. Appleton-Century-Crofts, New York, 1970, pp. 86-89.
11. Maigne, R.: Orthopedic Medicine. Charles C Thomas, Springfield, Ill., 1972, p. 379.
12. Bauwens, P., and Cayer, A.B.: The "multifidus triangle" syndrome as a cause of recurrent low back pain. Br. Med. J. 2:1306-1307, 1955.
13. King, J.S., and Lagger, R.: Sciatica viewed as a referred pain syndrome, in Surgical Neurology (in press).
14. Heyman, C.H.: The relief of low back pain and sciatica by release of fascia and muscle. J. Bone Joint Surg. 23:474-477, 1941.
15. Bensman, L.L., and Bensman, A.S.: Iliolumbar ligament syndrome: a frequent cause of low back pain. Arch. Phys. Med. Rehab. 59:11, 1978.
16. Bagley, C.E.: The articular facet in relation to low back pain and sciatic radiation. J. Bone Joint Surg. 25:481, 1941.
17. Kellgren, J.H.: On the distribution of pain arising from deep somatic structures with charts of segmental pain areas. Clin. Sci. 4:35, 1939.
18. Sinclair, D.C., Feindel, W.H., Weddell, J., and Falconer, M.A.: The intervertebral ligaments as a source of segmental pain. J. Bone Joint Surg. 30-B(3):515-521, 1948.
19. Rees, W.S.: Multiple bilateral subcutaneous rhizolysis of segmental nerves in the treatment of intervertebral disc syndrome. Ann. Gen. Prac. 26:126, 1974.
20. Pedersen, H.E., Blank, C.F.J., and Gardener, E.: Anatomy of lumbosacral posterior rami and meningeal branches of spinal nerves. J. Bone Joint Surg. 35-A:377, 1956.
21. Shealy, C.N., Prieto, A., Burton, C., and Long, D.M.: Radio frequency percutaneous rhizotomy of the articular nerve of Luschka—an alternative approach to chronic low back pain and sciatica. Paper presented to the American Association of Neurological Surgeons, Los Angeles, April 9, 1974.
22. Pere, E.R.: Mode of action of nociceptors, in Hirsch, C., and Zatterma, Y. (eds.): Cervical Pain. Pergamon Press, Oxford, 1972.
23. Steindler, A.: The interruption of sciatic radiation and the syndrome of low back pain. J. Bone Joint Surg. 22:28-34, 1948.
24. Steindler, A., and Luck, J.: Differential diagnosis of pain low in the back. J.A.M.A. 110:108-112, 1938.
25. Melzack, R., Stillwell, D.M., and Fox, E.J.: Trigger points and acupuncture points for pain: correlation and implication. Pain 3:3-23, 1977.
26. Maigne, R.: Charniere dorsolumbaire et lombalgier bases. Gaz. Med. France 85(11):1181-1194, 1978.
27. Maigne, R.: The concept of painlessness and opposite motion in spinal manipulations. Am. J. Phys. Med. 44(2):55-69.
28. Burton, C., and Nida, G.: Gravity lumbar reduction therapy program. Sister Kenny Institute Publication No. 731, 1976.

29. Nachemson, A.: The load on lumbar discs in different positions of the body. Clin. Orthop. 45:107-122, 1966.
30. Lindahl, O.: Hyperalgesia of the lumbar nerve roots in sciatica. Acta Orthop. Scand. 37:367-374, 1966.
31. Oudenhoven, R.C.: The role of laminectomy, facet rhizotomy and epidural steroids. Spine 4(2):145-147, 1979.
32. Dilke, T.F.W., Burry, H.C., and Graham, R.: Extradural corticosteroid injection in management of lumbar nerve root compression. Br. Med. J. 2:635-637, 1973.
33. Green, L.N.: Dexamethasone in the management of symptoms due to herniated lumbar disc. J. Neurol. Neurosurg. Psychiatry 38:1211-1217, 1975.
34. Burn, J.M.B., and Langdon, L.: Lumbar epidural injection for treatment of chronic sciatica. Rheumatol. Phys. Med. 10(7):368-374, 1974.
35. Hartman, J., Winnie, A.P., Ramaurthy, S., Mani, M.R., and Meyers, H.L.: Intradural and extradural corticosteroids for sciatic pain. Orthop. Rev. 3(12):21-24, 1974.
36. Goldie, I., and Peterhoff, V.: Epidural anesthesia in low back pain and sciatica. Acta Orthop. Scand. 39:261-269, 1968.
37. Gentry, W.D., Newman, M.C., Goldner, J.L., and von Breyer, C.: Relation between graduated spinal block technique and MMPI for diagnosis and prognosis of chronic low back pain. Spine 2(3):210-213, 1977.
38. Brena, J.F., and Unikel, I.P.: Nerve blocks and contingency management in chronic pain states, in Bonica, J.J., and Albe-Fessard, D. (eds.): Advances in Pain Research and Therapy. Vol. 1. Raven Press, New York, 1976.
39. Hirsch, C., Inglemark, B., and Miller, M.: The anatomic basis for low back pain. Acta Orthop. Scand. 33:1-17, 1963.

BIBLIOGRAPHY

Adams, J.E., and Inman, V.T.: Stretching of the sciatic nerve. Cal. Med. 91(1):24-26, 1959.
Anderson, T.P., Sachs, E., Fischer, R.G., and Kraut, R.M.: Postoperative care in lumbar disc syndrome. Arch. Phys. Med. Rehab. 42:152-158, 1961.
Doran, D.M.L., and Newell, D.J.: Manipulation in treatment of low back pain: a multicentre study. Br. Med. J. 26:161-164, 1975.
Parsons, W.B., and Boake, H.K.: Manipulation for backache and sciatica. Appl. Therapeutics 8(11):954-961, 1966.
Ray, M.B.: Manipulative treatment. Br. J. Phys. Med. 13(11):241-254, 1950.
Steer, J.C., and Horney, F.D.: Evidence for passage of cerebrospinal fluid along spinal nerves. Can. Med. Assoc. J. 98:71-74, 1968.

CHAPTER 5

Correction of Faulty Mechanics in Therapeutic Approach to Low Back Pain

After the acute phase of low back pain has subsided, the next phase of treatment is to prevent recurrence or to decrease residual pain and impairment. This phase requires

1. reconditioning the individual by regaining flexibility and strength;
2. retraining in proper bodily function to improve posture, occupational habits, and activities of daily living;
3. correcting or modifying psychosocial aspects of the individual's life.

Should the pain that was acute persist with objective neurologic deficits indicative of intervertebral disc herniation with nerve root entrapment, further evaluation and appropriate treatment must be undertaken.

If the acute pain persists with minimal organic findings that indicate possible evolution into *chronic pain*, further therapeutic approaches must be considered. All of these approaches should have been invoked in the acute phase but now require emphasis.

Should unusual or extraordinary conditions have been discovered during the acute phase of pain that portend to continued pain and disability, these require special study and care. These conditions include spinal stenosis, spondylolisthesis, arachnoiditis, and numerous other conditions mentioned in Chapter 8.

Any unusual condition obviously requires special diagnostic and therapeutic consideration, but there are basic concepts that pertain to any and all low back pain syndromes. These concepts must be considered in all patients complaining of low back pain.

FAULTY POSTURE CONCEPTS

The treatment of faulty posture causing static pain is fundamentally simple in its prescription. Insofar as faulty and painful posture is usually one of increased lordosis the treatment is to teach a *flat low-back* exercise. The increase in lordosis is dependent on the lumbosacral angle; therefore, the remedy is to change the pelvic angle. In essence *"tuck in the pelvis"* is the instruction.

The concept of the *tuck in* may be difficult for the patient to understand or feel. Since sway-back posture usually has been of long duration, the pattern is now well established. Even though lordotic posture will be causative of pain, this increase in lumbar arch *is* the *natural*, effortless postural pattern and in the patient there is likely inherent tendency to resist change, especially when effort and repeated effort must be made.

The factors that led to the original formation of this postural pattern are well established and are not easily broken. The familial tendency in the patient may frequently lead to a pessimism that "the condition runs in my family and is beyond my control." Minimal effort resulting in no immediate results may be sufficiently discouraging to some patients to end all further efforts. What is considered maximum effort for some patients is minimal cooperation for others, and vice versa. The constitutional variants and the psychologic factors that enter into cooperation can frequently tax the doctor. Serious questions concerning the correctness of diagnosis and prescribed treatment may arise in the mind of the doctor when the patient states, "I have done the exercises faithfully for months, and my back still hurts in the same way when I stand."

Adherence by the patient to his prescribed exercise program must be constantly and frequently supervised and reviewed. When these same exercises are later demonstrated to the doctor by the patient, it is amazing how distorted prescribed exercises may become a few weeks after the initial description by the doctor. The method or manner of doing these exercises may have no resemblance to that prescribed. Again, the reason for doing the exercises may frequently not be understood and must time and again be retaught. The addition of other exercises that neutralize the value of the prescribed regime occasionally are added by the patient himself. These neutralizing exercises are usually of the back-arching, hyperextension variety. Such exercises will be discussed in more detail in the section on exercises.

Probably the greatest failure occurs in the case of the patient who does his exercises faithfully but fails to "carry over" the posture to everyday activities. The performance of exercises is basically a training device and must be integrated into every activity of everyday living.

Posture is a full-time function of the body and must be maintained properly during every waking hour—standing, walking, sitting, in fact, in any upright stance. To exercise merely one hour a day every day and stand in a faulty manner the remainder of the 15 hours in which the patient is awake will lead to no improvement in posture and no decrease in pain.

For the patient whose posture is a portrayal of his emotional state there will obviously be little or no carry-over. In the chronically depressed person, more than exercise is needed. Drugs may help and even psychiatric intervention may be necessary. Such posture is the "picture" the patient wishes to portray to the world for his own psyche satisfaction; treatment from strictly mechanical-postural approach will fail.

Fatigue plays a large part in failure. In the psychasthenic person who does not possess a constitutional potential for endurance, no amount of exercise, drugs, or even corseting will give the necessary stamina, ligamentous tone, and muscle tone. The person does not have the resources, and as the muscle tone leaves the patient the ligaments become the only support and pain ensues.

There is the acceptable fatigue that occurs in everyone who reaches then exceeds his tolerance by hard work, prolonged activity, inadequate rest, or who is performing tasks for which he is anatomically or physically not suited. The problem in such instances is the recognition of these fatigue factors and the ability of the patient to make the necessary changes.

When the consideration of all these factors indicates that the problem is mechanical and demands flat-back treatment, pelvic-tilting exercises and their functional application must be taught and utilized.

LOW BACK STRETCHING EXERCISES

A tight low back, or inflexible lumbar spine, will impede trunk flexion. This condition may have been discovered during the examination when the physician observed the patient bending forward from the upright position. Stretch pain elicited on flexing of the tight lower back may have been determined to be the cause of the low back pain. If the inelasticity of the low back is present and symptomatic, it must be made elastic or flexible. The lumbar-spinal longitudinal ligaments and muscles must be stretched to regain this elongation range.

Normally a muscle contracts voluntarily, initiating no stretch reflex. This is mediated through neurologic reflexes within the cord. If there is "spasm" (i.e., a muscle contraction as a result of trauma or excessive abrupt stretch), the insult is to the intrafusal fibers initially and then to the extrafusal fibers (Fig. 75).

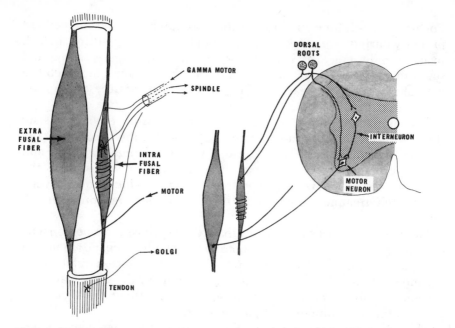

FIGURE 75. Intrafusal and extrafusal system. The extrafusal system consists of large muscle fibers under voluntary control. The intrafusal fibers consist of gamma motor neurons that "set" the muscle length for reflex action. The spindle cells report the muscle length and tension to the central nervous system. The Golgi neurons respond to the length and tension within the muscle tendon.

If the insult is moderate or severe, microscopic edema or hemorrhage can result that may persist as an irritating focus. This becomes a "trigger" zone or a so-called myofascial fibrositic nodule. The muscle remains contracted, thus refusing to elongate or "play out" during elongation.

Flexion of the lumbar spine is thus limited. The normal forward flexion allowed by reversal of the lordosis into lumbar kyphosis for the first 45 degrees of flexion is limited and can be painful. The spine assumes an "antalgic" posture. If the spasm is unilateral, a scoliosis results.

Persistence of this traumatic myofascial irritation may result in fibrous contracture and limited movement. Chronic pain may also result.

Acute pain, chronic pain, and anxiety with musculoskeletal manifestation can and do initiate the insult or injury that creates the ultimate vicious circle.

Prior to exercises, modalities of heat, ice, or cooling spray affect the spindle system to permit the muscles to "relax" and elongate. Exercises, both passive and active, must ultimately be utilized to elongate the muscles, fascia, and ligaments.

Low back stretching is best done initially in the "curled-up" or fetal

110

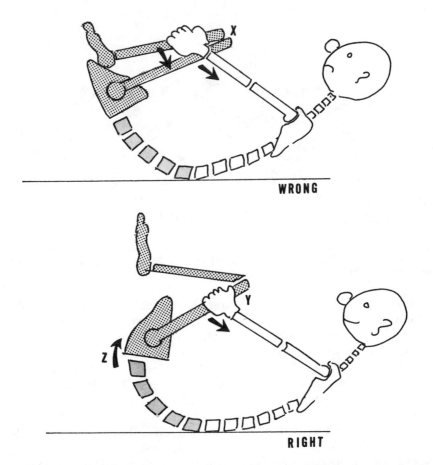

FIGURE 76. Low back flexibility exercises. The legs are used as a lever to flex the lumbar spine, as depicted in the lower drawing. The upper drawing shows the knees being hyperflexed, which stresses the knees without flexing the lower back.

position. This position, essentially a knee-to-chest position, is attempted so that the patient feels his low back being "stretched." The pelvis must be elevated from the floor or surface upon which the patient is lying supine. Merely flexing the knees to the chest does not necessarily flex the low back (Fig. 76).

Initially the knees must be brought to the chest by using both hands. Once the full available flexion has been attained, the gained position is held for a full minute or until it is felt that there is relaxation and elongation of the low back muscles. Further flexion can then be gained and again held. Finally full flexion can be achieved.

This gentle stretch and maintaining of full elongation of the erector spinae muscles serve to "unload" the spindle system, both intrafusal fiber spindles and the tendon Golgi apparatus (see Fig. 75).

111

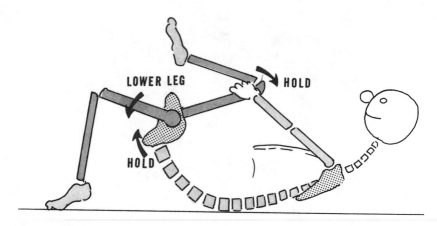

FIGURE 77. Descent from flexion exercise. After having flexed the low back to its maximum, *one* leg should be returned to the floor while maintaining a flexed pelvis. This prevents the return of lordosis during the descent of both legs, which may be painful.

As the erector spinae muscles (spinalis, longissimus, and iliocostals) attach along the thoracic vertebrae, the ribs and some fibers to the cervical spine *full flexion* should ultimately be gained.

Once the flexed position has been achieved, the legs can reextend slowly *one at a time.* To allow both legs to return to their extended position will frequently result in some extension of the low back. This sudden return of lordosis is often painful and can initiate spasm (Fig. 77).

By holding one knee flexed to the chest, the other leg can return to the floor without losing the gained lumbar kyphosis. The descending leg's return to the position of foot to the floor with flexed knee and hip is desired.

Insofar as the erector spinae muscle group is largely fascia, this tissue will need longer, gentle and progressive stretch even after relaxation of the muscle. (See discussion of the erector spinae muscle in Chapter 1.)

As the extensor muscles are unilateral, they must be laterally stretched. This can be done in the standing position with legs held apart. The knee on the side toward which the spine is laterally flexed may be flexed to insure greater elongation of the erector spinae muscles.

As the shoulder muscles attach to the ribs and to the spine and pelvis (trapezius and latissimus dorsi), they should also be elongated. This can be incorporated into the exercises by placing the arm overhead and toward the side of lateral motion (Fig. 78).

Manual stretching, as a part of manipulation or mobilization, undoubtedly benefits the patient because of muscle-fascial stretching. The concept of "Rolfing" is intended for this purpose. The recent

112

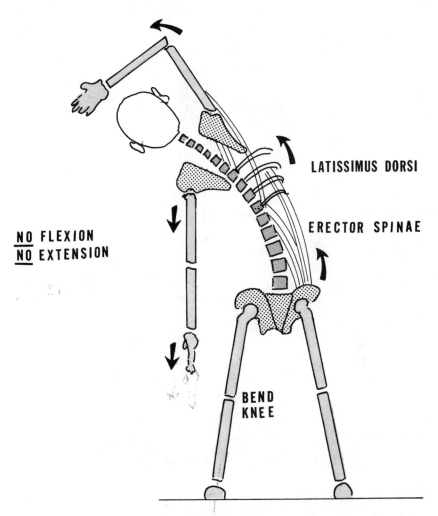

LATISSIMUS DORSI

ERECTOR SPINAE

<u>NO</u> FLEXION
<u>NO</u> EXTENSION

BEND
KNEE

FIGURE 78.   Lateral flexion exercises. With both legs apart slightly and one knee bent, the trunk is gently and progressively flexed laterally *without forward or backward flexion*. The unilateral erector spinae muscles and their fascia are stretched. As the scapular muscles also attach to stabilize the spine, they too must be stretched by placing the arms overhead.

development of gravity traction, in which gravity is applied to the body, also utilizes this principle (Fig. 79).

A modification of the supine low-back stretch is the *yoga* position. The patient sits with both knees flexed toward the chest and with knees spread apart sufficiently to permit the body to bend down between the separated knees. The head is "bobbed" down toward the feet. The feet may be grasped by the hands, the elbows being between the legs, to permit the arms to help stretch the lower back. This exercise is more

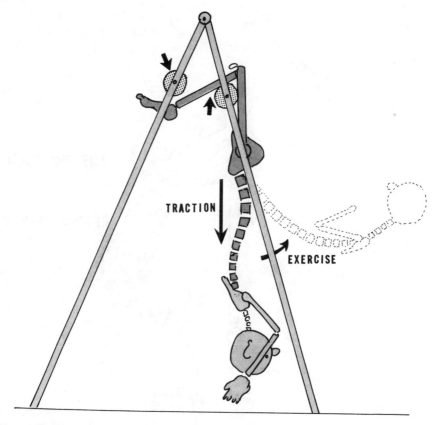

FIGURE 79. Gravity traction stretch exercises. By hanging from the lower extremities, the upper body weight applies traction to the spine. Lateral flexion can be achieved in this manner. Flexion exercises (*dotted lines*) strengthen the abdominal muscles.

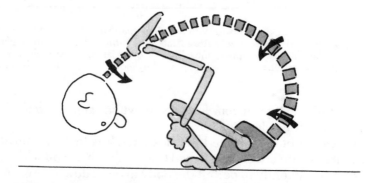

FIGURE 80. "Yoga" exercise. With the patient in a squat position, with the knees and hips flexed, the low back is gradually flexed until the head approaches the floor or the toes. This exercise fully stretches the entire spine.

114

taxing than that of the supine knee-to-chest exercise and will require careful supervision and a slower gradual increase (Fig. 80).

Any tendency to stretch the lower back by bending forward in an upright position with knees stiff, in a bouncing attempt to touch the toes with the fingers, should be initially avoided. This exercise can stretch the lower back but does so forcefully, inasmuch as the hamstrings hold the pelvis fixed after a certain degree of rotation. Because the hamstrings are less elastic and resilient, they do not "give" and impart the stretch upon the low back. The ability to bend forward and touch one's toes with the knees held extended is not a criterion of normal flexibility. As an exercise it may stretch the low back excessively.

PELVIC-TILTING EXERCISES

Initially, pelvic tilting is easier taught when the patient lies in a supine position. A firm surface upon which the patient lies supine is preferable to a soft surface, as it permits greater awareness of the points of body contact. After pelvic tilting has been mastered in a supine position, it must ultimately be performed in the upright position. The concept of this ultimate transition must be kept in mind from the onset.

The exercise is begun with the person lying supine in a comfortable position, hips and knees flexed, both feet flat on the floor, and the head relaxed on a pillow. In this position the first movement is that of the patient forcing or "pressing" his lower back down flat to the floor. This movement is performed by the combined contraction of the abdominal and the gluteal muscles, but the effect is "felt" by the patient in his hamstring and quadriceps muscles as well. A "squeezing" sensation of the hips and thighs is experienced. Placing the patient's hand at the "small" of the back and having him press down on his hand may help him in understanding the intended movement. A sharp object may be used beneath the back to give the patient an awareness of the proper feeling of the posture (Fig. 81).

A pillow under the patient's head will obviate any strain which may arise from stress in supporting the head or from improper breathing during the course of the exercise. Neck strain may become so distracting that it overshadows the concept of proper pelvic movement.

Once the lower back is pressing against the floor, the pelvis is rotated by raising the buttocks from the floor. Muscular effort is required for this movement. As the buttocks are being raised, the lower back *must not be permitted to leave the floor*. Allowing the low back to arise from the floor would be equivalent to a "wrestler's bridge." This would result in *hyperextension* of the lumbar spine rather than in the reversal of lordosis caused by raising the buttocks while the lower back is pressed flat against the floor.

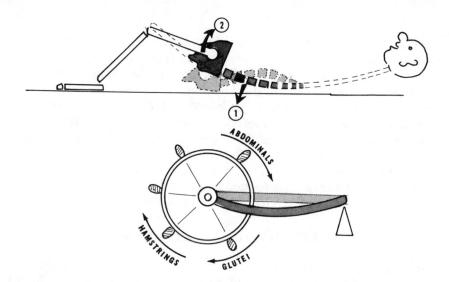

FIGURE 81. Concept of pelvic tilting. *Above:* (1) pressing the lumbar spine against the floor, table, or bed; (2) gentle gradual lifting of the pelvis from the floor or bed. *Below:* The musculature involved in pelvic tilting.

A helpful teaching tip is to place one hand on the symphysis pubic region, the other at the xiphoid process, and bring them together in the front, while the pelvis is elevated at the same time.

The patient is next taught slow rhythmic elevation of the pelvis with the lower back remaining *flat* against the floor. This permits smooth pelvic tilting which not only flattens the lumbar lordosis but gives the patient the kinesthetic concept of this tilting movement and simultaneously helps stretch the lower back. Endurance, as well as strength, is developed in the gluteal and abdominal muscles, which are the principal pelvic-tilting muscles.

As the concept and the ability to flatten the back is achieved with the hips fully flexed the attempt should now be made to continue the tilting movement while the legs are gradually extended. As the legs utlimately become fully extended, the upright position, or its equivalent, is assumed. Flattening of the lower back becomes increasingly more difficult as the legs become more extended at the hips. Any degree of tightness or restriction of the hip flexors increases the difficulty in flattening the lower back.

ERECT "FLAT BACK" EXERCISE

Standing up against a wall with both feet 6 to 12 inches away from the wall, the low back is pressed against the wall, then the pelvis (buttocks) is smoothly pulled away from the wall.

116

FIGURE 82. Erect pelvic tilting training. With the patient standing against a wall with feet slightly forward, the pelvis is "flattened" against the wall as it is against the floor in the supine exercise. This trains the patient to feel the position of the "flat" lumbar spine.

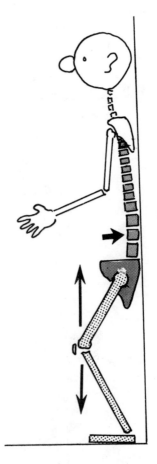

Progression of this exercise has the patient perform a series of slow deep-knee bends while keeping the pelvis "tilted." In essence the pressed area of the low back "slides" against the wall.

This exercise (1) teaches the concept of erect (upright) pelvic tilting, thus also teaching proper posture; (2) instructs the patient in bending with lumbar spine lordosis decreased; and (3) strengthens the quadriceps (knee extensors) that must be used in proper bending and lifting (Fig. 82).

Insofar as posture is a *concept* without specific cognizance of what specific muscles are doing, a method of achieving this postural concept has been developed by the author.

By supporting a moderately heavy weight on the head, pushing the weight upward, and standing *taller* to realign the body to the center of gravity, the cervical lordosis as well as the lumbar lordosis will be decreased[1] (Figs. 83 and 84).

117

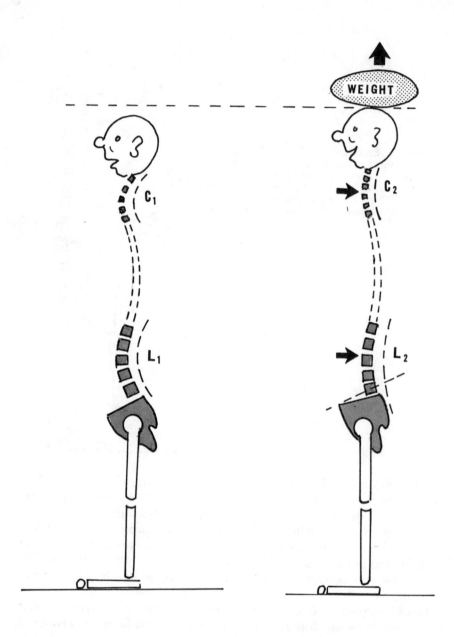

FIGURE 83. Erect posture concept training: *"distraction."* Placing a balanced weight upon the head and "pushing upward" (being taller) decreases the cervical and lordotic curves. The posture improves without the patient's awareness of any specific action of the pelvis or the shoulders. The "concept" of erect posture is gained unconsciously and can become habit.

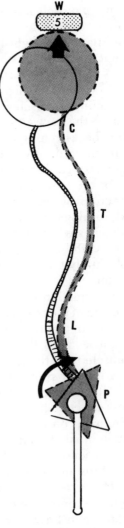

FIGURE 84. Mechanism of distraction exercise. By distracting the spine, elevating the weight upon the head, the cervical and lumbar curves decrease and the pelvis rotates.

By doing this exercise the *concept* of erect posture is achieved without concern about tucking in the pelvis or pulling back the shoulders, as these will "fall into place." By using this head weight for varying periods daily in standing, walking, and sitting, erect posture is maintained. Later, *without* the weight upon the head, the posture can be maintained. The weight can vary from 2 to 20 lbs, as tolerated and as needed by each individual patient.

ABDOMINAL STRENGTHENING EXERCISES

In a study of the muscular mechanism by which the pelvis is tilted, it is obvious that strength and endurance must exist in the abdominal and gluteal muscles. It is tempting for the patient knowing this to proceed on his own to develop his abdominal muscles by the classical exercise of bilateral straight-leg raising done while in the supine position. Except in extremely athletic and physically well-conditioned individuals, this exercise is *contraindicated.*

In view of the heaviness of the legs and the frequent weakness of the abdominal muscles, the first degrees of bilateral straight-leg raising cause the back to arch, and as a result the legs move very slightly. To this back-arching effect is added the intra-abdominal strain, plus the breath-holding Valsalva effect; therefore the contraindication to bilateral straight-leg raising from the supine position can be understood.

In the supine position, with both legs fully extended, the first 30 degrees of straight-leg raising is done by the iliopsoas muscle. The kinesiology of the ilipsoas muscle is hip flexion. The psoas muscle attaches within the abdomen from the anterolateral aspect of the lumbar vertebrae and their transverse processes. This muscle bundle obliquely traverses the pelvis to attach to the lesser trochanter of the femur.

Contraction of the iliopsoas on the fixed lumbar spine results in flexion of the femur on the pelvis. When the femur is fixed the converse occurs in that the psoas insertion becomes the origin, and the origin in turn becomes the insertion on the lumbar spine. Shortening of the muscle from the fixed femur causes traction on the anterior portion of the lumbar spine and results in increase in lumbar spine lordosis.

After 30 degrees or more of straight-leg raising, the iliopsoas becomes less effective in contraction and the abdominals become more efficient. From this position the pelvis will rotate and the lumbar spine flatten. If abdominal strengthening exercises are to be prescribed, they should begin when the legs have been raised to an angle of 30 degrees or when the hips and knees are flexed.

The *curl-up* from the supine position, with the hips and knees flexed, is the second stage of abdominal-muscle strengthening. *Curl-up* can be done from the supine position in which the head and shoulders are *peeled* up from the floor with a gradual curl to the point of having the nose touch the knees. This exercise requires strong abdominal muscles but may be done with the feet held down.

In the presence of significant weakness of the abdomen, this exercise can be done in reverse. The *curl-up* exercise is done as an *uncurl* exercise. From the fully curled-up position, with nose to knees, the patient leans back slightly from his flexed knees. After a few degrees of

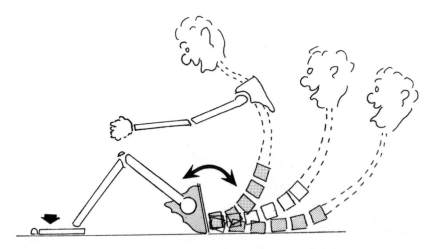

FIGURE 85. Abdominal flexion exercises from shortened position. Beginning in a full-flexed position, the body is gradually lowered, the postion sustained and returned to upright position, permitting full flexion gradually from supine position. Arms are held near knees to prevent excessive extension.

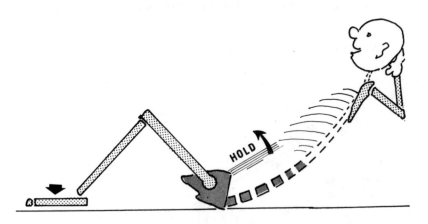

FIGURE 86. A partial flexed position used to strengthen pelvic muscles isometrically.

uncurling, the patient returns to the full-curled position. Progressive uncurling with return to full-flexed position is to be repeated until extension to the complete supine position and its return are possible (Figs. 85 and 86).

Intradiscal pressure studies have shown that there is less increase in intradiscal pressure during isometric abdominal exercises than is generated from isotonic exercises.

121

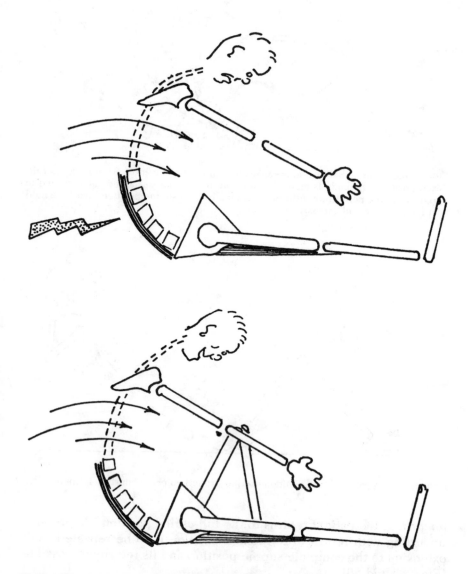

FIGURE 87. Protective hamstring stretching exercise. The upper drawing depicts the method of stretching both hamstrings simultaneously, which results in overstretching the low back. The lower drawing illustrates pelvic immobilization by flexing one hip and then stretching the other hamstring.

HAMSTRING STRETCHING EXERCISES

If the presence of tight hamstrings is discovered during the examination for flexibility, it is necessary that they be required to undergo stretching exercises. The inclination to stretch both hamstrings simultaneously by trying to bend forward at the trunk and keeping the legs extended may do harm, cause pain, and at best be ineffective as far as stretching the hamstrings is concerned. For this reason *protective* hamstring stretching is advocated (Fig. 87) the term *protective* implies that the low back is to be protected from excess stretching during the exercise.

The supine sitting position is used for the protective stretching exercise of the hamstring-muscle group. In such exercise the leg is fully flexed at the hip while the knee with the thigh is brought close to the chest; the foot in turn is placed flat against the floor. The leg undergoing the stretching exercise is extended straight ahead. Next, the flexed leg is rotated outward, and the knee is allowed to abduct. This action permits the patient to reach toward the toes of his extended leg. Reaching toward the toes is done in a bouncing, rhythmical manner. The stretch sensation must be felt in the extended leg. The flexed leg prevents stretching of the low back, and thus no pain from stretching can occur in the low back.

It must be kept in mind that this exercise is aimed at stretching connective tissue and myostatic contracture. If, however, the unilateral stretch pain is due to an irritable sciatic nerve rather than to inelastic connective tissue, this exercise will not be beneficial. As a rule, unilateral stretch pain emanating from straight-leg raising, with no contralateral stretch pain, more frequently is sciatica rather than pain caused by stretching tight hamstrings.

HEEL-CORD STRETCHING EXERCISES

When restrictive heel cords are found to impair body mechanics, they may be stretched during the course of the protective hamstring stretch-exercise by merely placing at a 90-degree angle the sole of the foot of the extended leg flat against a wall. The bouncing action which stretches the hamstring will simultaneously stretch the heel cord.

The heel cords may also be stretched effectively when the patient stands erect but leans forward against a wall. To take this position, the patient should stand a few feet away from the wall and stretch forward until the palms of his hands rest against the wall. In this position the body of the patient leans at an angle to the wall, but balanced on both feet and resting on both palms.

Once in this position, with *one* foot, the patient steps forward halfway

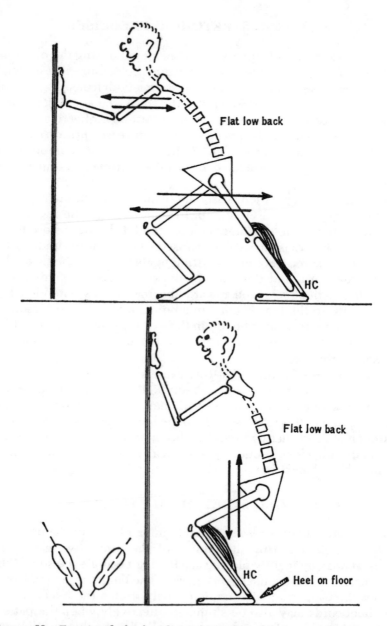

Flat low back

HC

Flat low back

HC Heel on floor

FIGURE 88. Exercises for heel cord stretching. The upper diagram illustrates the manner of stretching a bilateral heel cord by leaning against a wall and moving back and forth. The rear foot is kept flat against the floor, which insures stretching of the heel cord. The forward leg is flexed to permit to-and-fro rocking. The lumbar spine must be prevented from arching. In the lower diagram bilateral heel cord stretching is performed by squatting and sitting on both heels. The feet are placed slightly apart and externally rotated. The stretching motion is a rhythmic up-and-down bounce with balance maintained against a wall or chair.

to the wall. Keeping his other leg extended at the knee and the heel firmly on the ground, the patient then flexes rhythmically the forward leg at the knee. Flexing the arms allows a total back-and-forth movement of the entire body but the rear heel must be kept flat against the floor. In this way, a stretching effect is exerted on the heel cord (Fig. 88). Care must be taken during this exercise to prevent arching of the lower region of the back as the leaning position against the wall is conducive to arching. A flat back must be maintained constantly.

A method of bilateral heel cord stretching may be suggested (Fig. 88, lower portion) that appears exceedingly simple, yet cannot be performed by everyone. The person squats as if he intends to sit on his heels, and at the same time keeps both feet slightly turned out and several inches apart. Both heels must be kept on the floor and any use of the soles of the feet or toes must be avoided while a bouncing deep-knee bend is performed. In assuming the position necessary for this exercise the person will naturally feel the stretching taking place in heel cords. Because this exercise may place a person off balance, it should be done with support from a chair or wall.

EXERCISES FOR STRETCHING HIP FLEXORS

Stretching of tight hip flexors (the iliopsoas group) is a difficult exercise. The hip flexors are difficult to isolate and the stretching of hip flexors without simultaneously hyperextending the lumbar spine takes a concentrated effort; frequently it requires assistance. The correct stretching of this muscle group presupposes that the patient has mastered pelvic tilting and therefore is capable of maintaining a flat back during the exercise.

This exercise can be performed in several ways. One of them is done in the supine position with the extended leg held down against the floor. The extended leg is the one in which the hip flexor is to be stretched. This leg can be held down by placing the leg under a bed or sofa, by using a heavy sandbag, or by having another person render assistance. The opposite leg is then flexed rhythmically to the chest as in the knee-chest exercise.

As the flexed leg is brought repeatedly to the chest, the hip flexors of the opposite leg receive the benefit of the exercise.

In another form of the exercise, the patient may lie supine on a table or bed and dangle one leg from the table. The leg will then come into play to stretch the hip flexor. In this exercise there will also occur the stretching of the quadriceps femoris which may be prevented by reducing the degree of knee flexion of the dangling leg. The remainder of this exercise is done in the same manner as when it is performed on the floor (Fig. 89).

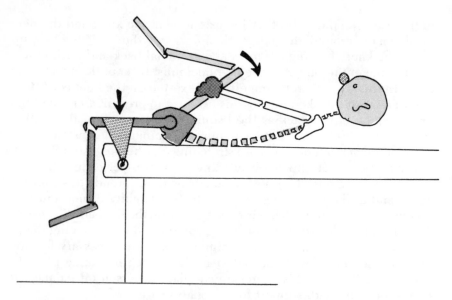

FIGURE 89. Hip flexor stretching exercise. With the hip held down, flexing the opposite hip to the chest tilts the pelvis and stretches the opposite hip flexor.

Unfortunately, tight hip flexors are very difficult to reextend to full hip extension. The daily habits of most people have them flexed during long periods of the day: sitting in cars, sitting at work, sitting at home, and lying supine or on their sides in the flexed position.

It is mandatory that if the hip flexors are to be kept extended, the patient must spend much of the day standing erect and lying prone at night without extending the low back.

BRACING AND CORSETING

Occasionally a patient who is convalescing from an episode of acute low back pain or who has had recurrent low back episodes will benefit from the use of a corset. A properly fitted corset or brace can be expected to

1. decrease the need for muscle "spasm" to splint the back for comfort during healing;
2. "unload" the lumbar spine by increasing the abdominal pressure when abdominal muscle tension is not possible;
3. improve the posture;
4. minimize movement of the lumbar spine, forcing any flexion to occur at the pelvis.[2,3]

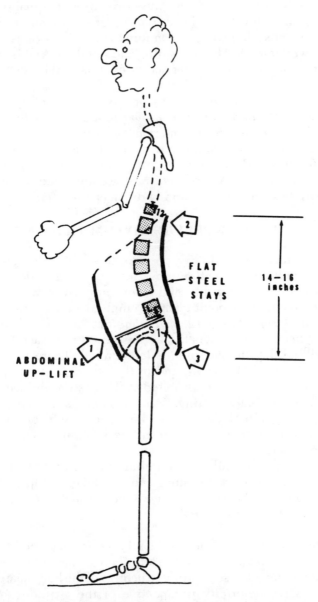

FIGURE 90. Corseting. Proper back support is based on three points of contact: (1) firm, uplifting abdominal support; (2) contact at the thoracolumbar junction; and (3) contact over the sacrum. Points 2 and 3 insure that the lumbar curve is "flat," indicating that lordosis is decreased.

To afford all these benefits, the corset must be properly fitted. It must be of adequate length, extending from the sacrum to the lower thoracic spine. Stays may be inserted posteriorly to influence a physiologic curving with minimal lordosis. Anteriorly the abdominal support must compress and elevate the lower portion of the abdomen (Fig. 90).

No corset fits adequately or comfortably in all positions. No corset is equally well tolerated both in sitting and standing. As it is most beneficial for standing and walking activities, this is the best position for fitting.

The corset may be fitted and worn by the patient upon becoming ambulatory. *It must, however, be worn as a means to an end* for a minimal duration to afford comfort and encourage activity and to minimize excessive lumbar spine movement. It must have a limited period of use to prevent disuse atrophy, myofascial contracture, and phychological dependence. A corset *must* be accompanied by simultaneous exercises, posture training, and body mechanics training.

LUMBAR-PELVIC RHYTHM TRAINING

All the exercises of flexibility, posture, and pelvic tilting will be of *no practical value* if the patient does not put them to daily use. If the patient does not bend, lift, and stoop properly, low back pain will probably recur. This point must be emphasized as *these instructions are the most important aspects of rehabilitating the low back patient.*

A *flat back* is so designated because the lumbosacral angle is decreased and the lumbar spine is less curved. There is less shearing stress of L_5 on S_1, L_4 on L_5, and in the others in the sequence. The posterior articulations are separated by this posture and accordingly are less subject to weight bearing. Less ligamentous strain is imposed and consequently better balance exists between muscle tone and ligamentous balance. All these factors insure less fatigue because of a better balanced spine.

Flat back posture fulfills the definition of correct body posture as described in the work "Posture and Its Relationship to Orthopedic Disabilities," by the Posture Committee of the American Academy of Orthopedic Surgeons in 1947:

> Posture is usually defined as the relative arrangement of the parts of the body. Good posture is the state of muscular and skeletal balance which protects the supporting structures of the body against injury or progressive deformity irrespective of the attitude (erect, lying, squatting, stooping) in which these structures are working or resting. Under such conditions the muscles will function most efficiently and the optimum positions are afforded for the thoracic and abdomi-

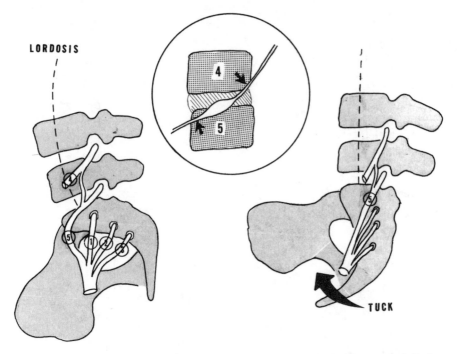

FIGURE 91. Relationship of lumbosacral plexus to lordosis. In the drawing at left, the lumbar lordosis has an angled L_5 root, owing to its attachment to the sacrum. With decrease of the lordosis, the L_5 root straightens and thus is under less tension.

nal organs. Poor posture is a faulty relationship of the various parts of the body which produce increased strain on the supporting structures and in which there is less efficient balance of the body over the base of support.

Likewise, in any kinetic operation of the body, a similarly balanced relationship of the parts to each other must remain to insure minimal strain and minimal muscular effort. Hence, during movement a flat back balanced over the plumb-line center of gravity should be maintained.

Throughout the discussion of erect static lumbar posture, the intent is to decrease the lordosis. In addition to discal effect, intradiscal pressures, and the length of the spinal canal, the angulation of the lumbosacral plexus is influenced.

In the straight lumbar curve with maximal lordosis, the fifth lumbar root (L_5) is curved and under no tension. In a lordotic posture the fifth lumbar root (L_5) is angulated by being attached to the ala of the sacrum.[4] Straight-leg raising and forward flexion place traction upon this root (Fig. 91).

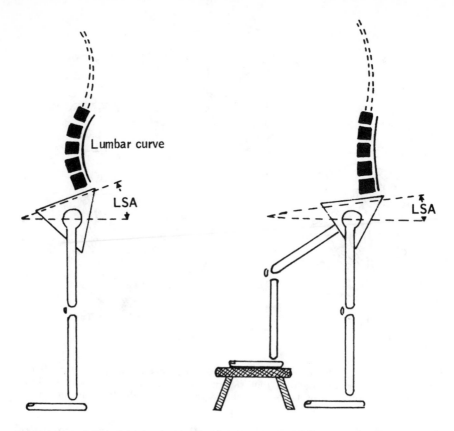

FIGURE 92.   Relaxed, prolonged standing posture. A small foot stool enables the hip of one leg to be flexed, thus relaxing the iliopsoas and "flattening" the lumbar curve. This method is advisable for dentists, housewives, and barbers, among others.

When the patient bends forward, the lumbar curve must reverse. It is necessary that the patient should learn to bend with his knees slightly flexed. In this way, the hamstrings are relaxed and, therefore, impose less restriction on pelvic rotation. This affords less occasion for forcing flexion of the lumbar spine beyond its physiologic limits.

For the person who must remain in a partially bent position during long periods of the day, such as the barber, dentist, or housewife who works over a sink or a crib, less fatigue will result from such posture if the back is kept flat and the center of gravity maintained over the hips and feet. No discomfort occurs in the absence of ligamentous strain.

Flexing one hip will help in assuming flat back posture by releasing hip-flexor pull on the lumbar spine. Thus, placing one foot on a small stool with the knee and hip flexed will permit an upright position with less lumbar lordosis (Fig. 92).

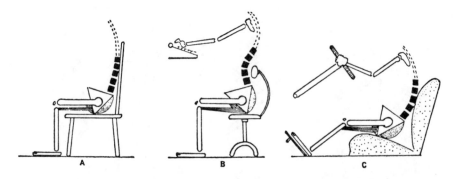

FIGURE 93. Sitting postures. A. Correct sitting posture in a firm, straight-back chair in which the seat has the proper width and height to allow hips and knee to be flexed with no strain and with both feet touching the floor. The back of the chair supports the low back 4 to 6 inches from the seat and permits a "flat" lumbar curve. B. The chair back increases the arch and causes a hamstring strain and a fatiguing low back posture. C. The hamstrings are taut and place traction on the pelvis, causing rotation and ultimately strain on the low back.

In everyday activities one must always keep in mind the benefit of a low back kept *flat*. In addition, all the tissues having a stressful reaction on the spine are kept inoperative. For example, neutral position of sitting erect in a pain-free effortless attitude requires a chair with a firm seat and back. The height of the seat should permit the legs to be flexed free at the knees. The base of the spine should rest merely a few inches forward of the chair back. The feet should reach the floor from a seat height that supports the thighs. When the rest of the chair is high, the feet may dangle placing pressure on the posterior thigh area and disrupt a relaxed pelvic balance. Too low a chair seat increases the hip flexor angle and forces a person to bend forward upon his pelvis. The chair back should offer firm contact for the spine 4 to 6 inches above the seat and an area of contact with the upper lumbar spine and the lower thoracic spine. This firm, flat chair-back permits the lumbar spine to be erect but prevents a fatiguing stance that is flexed so much it causes prolonged ligamentous strain.

In Figure 93, proper chair-sitting posture is illustrated in A. In the secretarial chair depicted in B, the support for the small of the back is too high and too narrow. The point of low-back contact is at the mid-lumbar point, forcing the spine to arch around this pressure fulcrum. The rotation of the pelvis resulting from this increased lordosis places a stretch strain on the hamstring muscles. The conflict between the hamstring pull and low-back arch terminates in fatigue and pain.

The automobile seat or the soft, deep sofa places an elongation hamstring pull on the pelvis with a resultant flexion on the lumbar

131

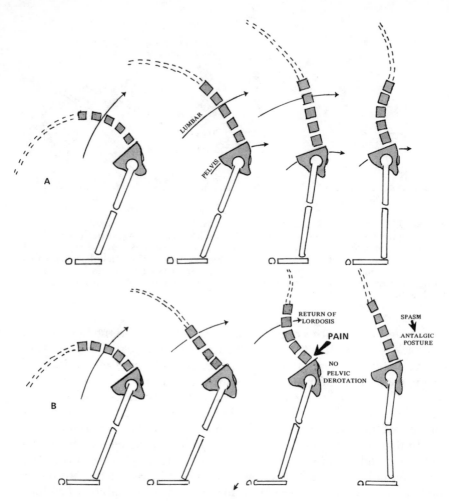

FIGURE 94. Proper vs. improper flexion and reextension. *A* depicts proper simultaneous resumption of the lumbar lordosis with pelvic rotation. *B* reveals the regaining of pelvic lordosis with no pelvic derotation, thus causing painful lordotic posture with the upper part of the body held ahead of the center of gravity.

spine that exceeds the flat lumbar curve. Pain in this instance arises from hamstring stretch and concurrent low-back posterior-longitudinal ligamentous strain.

PROPER BENDING AND LIFTING

Proper body mechanics implies proper bending forward and returning to the erect posture. This movement is done many times in the average day and consists of the motion of lifting, whether utilized in lifting a

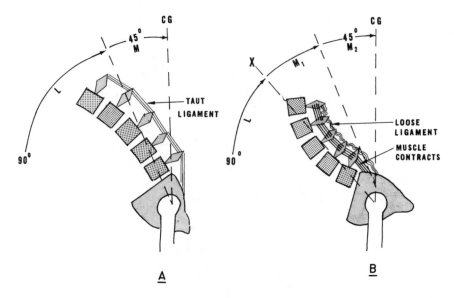

FIGURE 95. Faulty reextension of lumbar spine. *A.* Correct reextension. Until the last 45 degrees, the lumbar spine is supported (L) by supraspinous ligaments requiring no muscular effort. Muscles normally become active in the last 45 degrees (M) when the carrying angle is close to the center of gravity (CG). *B.* Premature lumbar lordosis with pelvis not adequately derotated causes the erector muscles (M_1) to contract before having reached the last 45 degrees. The ligaments loosen, and the muscles take the brunt and contract inefficiently and forcefully, resulting in pain.

heavy object, a light object, a bulky object, an object lifted from the floor or from waist level. *Improper bending and reassuming erect posture is probably the greatest cause of low back pain, with or without concomitant radicular pain.* No greater emphasis can be placed on any aspect of the mechanism of low back pain than on this fact.

The lumbar pelvic rhythm has been discussed. Faulty reextension from the flexed position, in which the lordosis is regained before the pelvis is derotated, is a major causative factor in low back pain (Fig. 94). This regains lordosis with the upper portion of the body in front of the center of gravity. Thus there is all the stress of hyperextension as in the static lordotic posture plus the extra extensor muscle contraction to maintain this cantilevered position.

Normally, the lumbar spine is supported by the supraspinous ligaments when in full flexion to extension until the last 45 degrees. The reextension to full erect posture is by pelvic derotation. For the last 45 degrees of extension the erector spinae muscles straighten the spine and regain the lordosis. Due to the short lower arm to which the erector spinae muscles are attached, this portion of reextension is inefficient (Fig. 95).

133

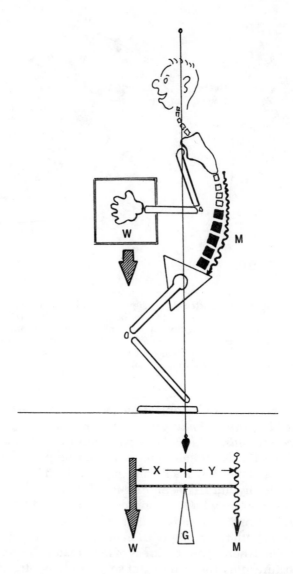

FIGURE 96. The relationship of the distance of a carried weight from the center of gravity and the resultant tension on the spinal musculature is expressed by the equation $W \times X = M \times Y$, where W = the weight of the object carried; X = the distance the weight is held from the center of gravity; Y = the distance of the spinal musculature from the center of gravity; and M = the tension developed by the musculature. In a simple lever system the weight supported by the fulcrum (G) is the sum of the weights acting at each end of the lever bar: 100×10 inches = 100×10 inches, thus G = 200 lbs; 100×20 inches = 200×10 inches, thus G = 300 lbs.

In faulty reextension in which the lordosis is regained prematurely with the upper body ahead of the center of gravity, this inefficient erector spinae muscle action upon the lumbar spine is made to support the body and perform further extension. This results in painful muscular contraction.

If the muscles fail to complete the function of reextension, the stress now falls acutely upon the extended (relaxed) ligaments.

As the facets separate during forward flexion, some rotation is possible in the cantilevered position. With rotation there is rotatory torque on the functional unit that is resisted mostly by the annular fibers. As a result some of these fibers can be torn (see Chapter 6).

Proper bending forward and reextending require coordinated lumbar flexion and return to the erect lordosis with simultaneous pelvic derotation. Also, with reextension to the erect posture there must be coordinated derotation in the sagittal plane if there has been any rotation in the fully flexed position.

If the purpose of bending and reextending has been to lift an object, either light or heavy, that object must be brought close to the body (Figs. 96, 97, and 98).

In lifting any object, the last 45 degrees of extension are accomplished by the erector spinae muscles but primarily by the tensed lumbar fascia and the extensor muscles of the pelvis. The shorter the distance the weight is to the center of gravity, the less muscular effort is required of the back extensor muscles.

Bringing the object that is being lifted closer to the body improves the efficiency of the short fulcrum arm of the posterior elements of the functional unit acting against the long lever of the arms and the lifted object (Fig. 99).

During the initial phase of lifting a heavy object there is need of increased abdominal tension and interabdominal pressure. This pressure is assumed to press posteriorly against the lumbosacral fascia to make this fascia taut. The taut fascia reinforces the strength and efficacy of the lumbar spine by relieving the stress upon the muscles and ligaments.

The sacrospinales muscle attaches to the lumbosacral fascia and acts to increase the tautness of the fascia (Fig. 100).

In reassuming the erect posture, until the last 45 degrees of extension is reached, the lumbar spine, being flexed, acts mechanically as an inflexible rod returning to the erect upon the rotating pelvis. The combination of the fascia, supraspinous ligaments, and the erector muscles gives this support. From 45 degrees of flexion to full erect stance the erector spinae muscles further extend the spine.

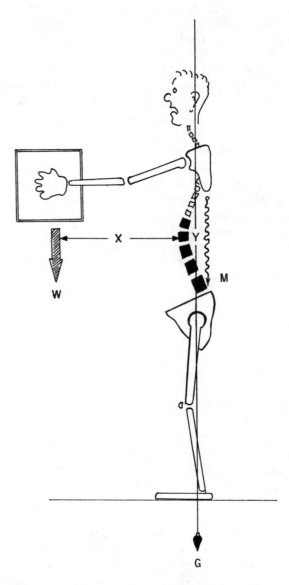

FIGURE 97. The increase of strain imposed upon the erect spine when an object of the same weight is held at arm's length. Using the formula $W \times X = M \times Y$, if $W = 100$ lbs, $X = 24$ inches, and $Y = 6$ inches, then $100 \times 24 = M \times 6$; thus $M = 400$ lbs, and $M + W = 500$ lbs. By increasing any component of a simple lever arm, the total weight superimposed on the supporting structure can be altered. Either changing the weight of the object held or increasing the distance from the body will increase the gravity (G) strain and will concurrently increase the muscular stress (M) as the distance (Y) changes little if at all. The M stress is a muscular compressive force on the vertebral discs.

136

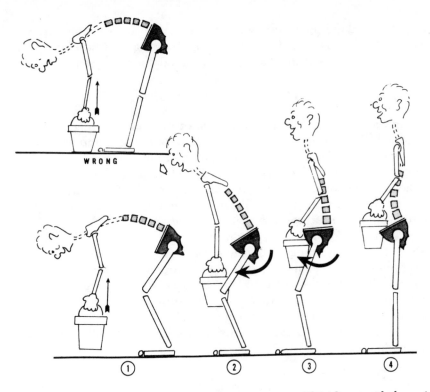

FIGURE 98. Proper method of lifting. The wrong way to lift is shown with the weight ahead of the body and the legs straight, causing strain. In proper lifting (lower drawing) the weight is brought close to the body while the pelvis tilts. The lumbar spine then gradually resumes the erect lordosis upon the tilted pelvis.

Proper bending forward and lifting must become a proper bodily movement that requires:

1. good flexibility of the low back and lower extremities;
2. good abdominal muscle tone;
3. good elongation and strength of the erector spinae muscles;
4. proper knowledge of the body mechanics, which requires:
   a. training,
   b. practice to make that action automatic,
   c. no distraction to impede its proper execution, which can result from
      (1) fatigue,
      (2) anxiety,
      (3) haste,
      (4) depression,
      (5) anger.

It is apparent that impairment with resultant pain and dysfunction can thus result from inadequate conditioning, training, and psychological distraction. Treatment must keep all these components in mind.

INTRADISCAL PRESSURE

Although many other factors must be kept in mind in explaining the physiology of the back in relation to posture, movement and exercises, recent studies of intradiscal pressures of the lumbar spine have added to current knowledge. The original studies of intradiscal pressure were related to static positions. Later studies concerned various movements as well as further static postures. These have been valuable in understanding specific postures, activities, and therapeutic exercises both in terms of assessing cause or aggravation of low back pain and in evaluating the physiologic efficacy of prescribed exercises.

Complete reliance on intradiscal pressures, currently reasonably well established, does not take into consideration muscular or ligamentous stresses as well as shear forces or torque forces. Nevertheless, intradiscal pressures have practical clinical value.

Approximate load measured on the L_3 disc (in a 70-kg individual) has been estimated as follows:[5]

Supine in traction	10 kg
Supine	30 kg
Erect with corset	30 kg
Erect standing	70 kg
Walking	85 kg
Twisting (erect)	90 kg
Bending sideways	95 kg
Upright sitting with no support	100 kg
Isometric abdominal exercises	110 kg
Coughing	110 kg
Jumping	110 kg
Straining	120 kg
Laughing	120 kg
Bending forward 20 degrees	120 kg
Bilateral straight leg raising in supine position	120 kg
Hyperextension exercise (prone)	150 kg
Sit-up exercises (knee extended)	175 kg
Sit-up exercises (supine with knees bent)	180 kg
Bending forward 20 degrees with 10 kg	185 kg
Lifting 20 kg with back straight and knees bent	210 kg
Lifting 20 kg with back bent but knees straight	340 kg

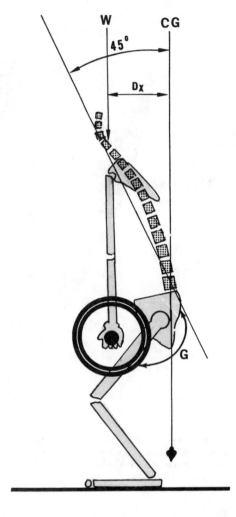

FIGURE 99. Heavy weight-lifting. With the weight close to the body (D_x) the fulcrum is more efficient. The muscles of the back (erector spinae) contract to elevate the spine during the last 45 degrees of extension. Until 45 degrees the fascia and ligaments of the lumbar spine carry the burden with the pelvic muscles rotating the pelvis.

These studies indicate that traction decreases intradiscal pressure and that a corset with an inflated abdominal pressure returns the pressure to the same as supine position, thus in part explaining the value of a corset (Fig. 101).

The low intradiscal pressure of walking explains why patients suffering low back pain often make the claim that they can walk (85 kg) but not sit (100 kg), why jogging is painful (110 kg), and why merely bending forward 20 degrees, as in many household activities (120 kg), is avoided.

In prescribing exercises it should be remembered that isometric

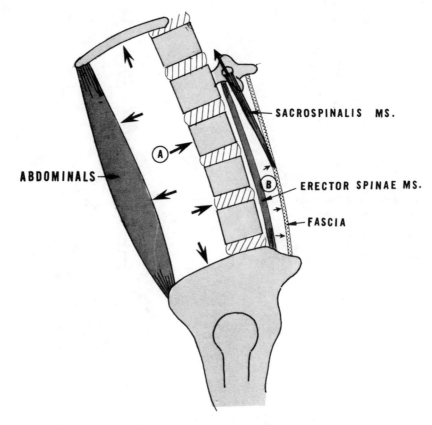

FIGURE 100. Increase in abdominal tension causes pressure posteriorly against the dorsolumbar fascia, causing it to become tense and thus relieving the tension upon the erector spinae muscles. The sacrospinalis muscle, by its attachment to the fascia, also increases its tension.

abdominal exercises (110 kg) are better tolerated than isotonic exercises (175-180 kg), regardless of knees being bent or straight.

In teaching proper bending and lifting techniques, the value of having a straight back with knees bent (210 kg), rather than lifting with the back and keeping knees straight (340 kg), is evident.

Nachemson's studies implied that the increase in tension was muscular rather than an increase in spinal fluid pressure.[6]

In studies done to test the effect of traction, 60 percent of the body weight as the traction force was needed to decrease lumbar intradiscal pressure.

Compression of abdominal contents "unloads" the lumbar spine.[7,8] This was studied by measuring intradiscal pressure with and without

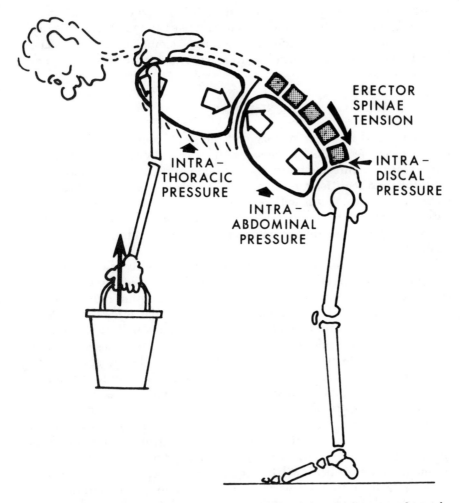

ERECTOR
SPINAE
TENSION

INTRA-
THORACIC
PRESSURE

INTRA-
DISCAL
PRESSURE

INTRA-
ABDOMINAL
PRESSURE

FIGURE 101. Abdominal-thoracic support of the spine. The intrathoracic and intraabdominal pressures created during the act of lifting decrease the pressure exerted by stress forces upon the intervertebral discs. This substantiates the efficacy of a corset, a brace with an abdominal support, and the need for strong abdominal muscles to insure a strong back.

an inflated corset with an abdominal pad. After inflating the abdominal pad, the pressure within the lumbar disc decreased to the degree measured in the supine position. Thus it was shown that an increase in abdominal pressure decreases the intradiscal pressure.

In lifting a heavy object from the floor there is a definite increase in abdominal pressure. In the Lamy-Farfan model the abdominal pressure is considered to be exerted posteriorly against the dorsolumbar fascia, causing the fascia to become taut. The tension upon the liga-

141

ments and the contracted extensor muscles is then decreased.[9]

The manner for doing abdominal exercises ranges from "sit-ups" (isotonic) to isometric abdominal exercises. Isometric exercises have been found to increase intradiscal pressure to a lesser extent than do isotonic exercises.

SUMMARY

As established from the history and physical examination, the treatment of the mechanical low-back pain is based on the correction of faulty *static* posture and faulty *kinetic* mechanism of the lumbar spine.

Static abnormalities are essentially the result of faulty posture, and correction of these faults with resultant good posture should result in a pain-free stance. Adequate flexibility, good muscle tone, and proper concept of good kinesthetics are essential for the maintenance of proper posture.

Proper *kinetic* function requires adequate flexibility of all movement components involved in the performance of correct *lumbar-pelvic rhythm*. All the components concerned in the rhythm must function correctly. Insofar as movement requires muscular effort, sometimes strength, and sometimes endurance, and at times both, good muscle conditioning is paramount. All factors composing the kinetic function must be adequate and must be organized in a facile and almost automatic functional pattern. Exercises will achieve maximum flexibility and produce maximum muscle strength and endurance. Proper performance constantly practiced will result in everyday function free of pain, owing to the proper use of a properly conditioned machine.

In spite of proper function resulting from instruction and judicious practice that insures normal body mechanics, any emotional or environmental interference, such as anger, impatience, depression, or anxiety, can cause faulty body use. The resultant pain and impairment can aggravate all the inciting factors, creating a vicious circle.

Proper static and kinetic function of the back is nearly always considered in conjunction with the psychological, social, and environmental influences on the patient.

REFERENCES

1. Jonck, L.M.: The influence of weight bearing on the lumbar spine: a radiological study. S. Afr. J. Radiol. 2(2):25-29, 1964.
2. Morris, J.M., and Lucas, D.B.: Biomechanics of spinal bracing. Arizona Med. March 1964, pp. 170-176.
3. Morris, J.M., Lucas, D.B., and Breslan, B.: Role of the trunk in stability of the spine. J. Bone Joint Surg. 43-A(3):327-351, 1961.
4. Goodard, M.D., and Reid, J.D.: Movements induced by straight leg raising in the lumbosacral roots, nerves and plexus, and on the intrapelvic section of the sciatic nerve. J. Neurol. Neurosurg. Psychiatry 28:12-18, 1965.

5. Nachemson, A.: Pathophysiology and treatment of back pain, in Buerger, A.A., and Tabis, J.S. (eds.): Approaches to the Validation of Manipulation Therapy. Charles C Thomas, Springfield, Ill., 1977.
6. Nachemson, A., and Elfstrom, G.: Intravital dynamic pressure measurements in lumbar discs. Scand. J. Rehab. Med. (Suppl. 1), 1970.
7. Bartelink, D.L.: The role of abdominal pressure in relieving the pressure on the lumbar intervertebral discs. J. Bone Joint Surg. 39-B:718-725, 1957.
8. Nachemson, A., and Morris, J.M.: In vivo measurements of intradiscal pressure. J. Bone Joint Surg. 46-A(5):1077-1092, 1964.
9. Gracovetsky, A., Farfan, H.F., and Lamy, C.B.: A mathematical model of the lumbar spine using an optimized system to control muscles and ligaments. Orthop. Clin. North Am. 8(1):135-153, 1977.

BIBLIOGRAPHY

Davis, P.R.: Posture of the trunk during lifting of weights. Br. Med. J. 1:87-89, 1959.
Keegan, J.: Alterations of the lumbar curve related to posture and seating. J. Bone Joint Surg. 35-A:589, 1953.
Knutsson, B., Lindh, K., and Telbag, H.: Sitting—an electromyographic and mechanical study. Acta Orthop. Scand. 37:415-428, 1966.

CHAPTER 6

Disc Disease

Disc disease today is considered to be a specific disease entity and the basic cause of most mechanical low back pain syndromes. The concept of disc disease unfortunately does not enjoy universal acceptance by the various medical specialties that are entrusted with the care of the patient with low back pain. Terms such as disc degeneration, rupture, slipping, bulging, and herniation are used indiscriminately to explain all symptoms of pain in the low back with or without radiation of pain into the lower extremity.

Much is known concerning the anatomy and chemistry of the intervertebral disc. The physiology is becoming understood and its pathophysiology better defined. Sufficient knowledge is had today to interpret its normal function and to evaluate its deviation from normal. The basis for pain is becoming clearer as is the neurologic aspect of disability. Chronic pain in the low back sufferer may someday be decreased as the acute, recurrent, and persistent episodes are better evaluated and treated. A rational therapeutic approach is gradually emerging.

The intervertebral disc is a hydraulic system composed of a fibro-elastic envelope containing a colloidal gel in its center. This nucleus has definite intrinsic pressure that maintains the separation of the vertebral bodies so that the functional unit retains its stability and its mobility.

The intervertebral disc is the predominant portion of the functional unit and any defect, injury, or degenerative change will, and does, change the dynamics of the unit. All pain and impaired function, however, are not specifically or uniquely related to disc disease. Its place in the low back syndrome must be clearly and carefully evaluated and ascertained.

LUMBAR DISC HERNIATION

Disc herniation is fundamentally a release of the nuclear material from the confinement of the enveloping annulus fibrosus capsule. Herniation of the nuclear material may result from excessive forces, repeated stresses, and prolonged tension on the hydraulic mechanism or the presence of a faulty annulus, but any combination of the above may be involved. The formula previously mentioned may be applied here and the solution sought for in (1) abnormal stress on normal mechanism, (2) normal stress on an abnormal mechanism, or (3) normal stress on a normal mechanism when the mechanism is not prepared to accept the stress.

Compressive forces applied directly to the functional unit will cause vertebral body compression before any disc disruption of the intact disc. Rotational forces, however, place torque upon the annular fibers which become disrupted, and the intradiscal nuclear pressure is no longer contained.[1] This central pressure forces the encircling annular fibers outward to encroach upon pain-sensitive tissues, such as the posterior longitudinal ligament and the nerve root and its dura (Fig. 102).

On a purely mechanical basis the outer annular fibers having greater torque in rotational movements tear first.[2] By being close to surrounding sensitive ligamentous tissues, they can cause pain when they tear. Due to mechanical factors[3] there is greater intradiscal pressure in the posterior lateral quadrants of the disc where the pain-sensitive tissue of the neural canal is located. Fibers in these quadrants are more prone to give under pressure.

Lumbar disc herniation is unquestionably a specific disease entity. The term *herniation,* or *rupture,* is more explainable and understandable in a mechanical sense than the term *slipped. Bulging* of the disc is also an accepted term. It is sufficient to say that the term used is of less importance than the realization of what is happening. It is much more significant to know the *where* and *what* of the disc herniation that is causing the symptoms, the *why* of the consequent treatment, and the *when* if there is a need for surgical intervention. The complete *why* or the course of the disc rupture is not yet understood fully.

Symptoms

Clinically the patient who sustains a disc herniation presents a history of acute low back pain with or without sciatic radiation. *Sciatica* is generally understood to mean referred pain or hyperaesthesia—paresthesia or dyasthesia down the course of the involved nerve root. The patient may describe this discomfort as "burning," "aching," "sharp,"

145

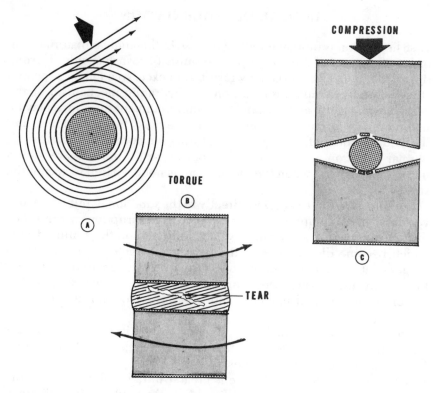

FIGURE 102. Compression versus torque effect upon annulus. *A.* Annular fibers. Because the outer fibers are longer and more distant from the axis of rotation, they sustain greater torque force in rotation (*arrow*) and thus can tear more easily (*B*). *C.* Compression force can damage the vertebral body before damaging the disc. The endochondral plates can be penetrated by the nucleus.

"dull," or "tender." The sensation may be localized by the patient as being across the low back, into the buttocks, along the posterior-lateral thigh, along the calf, or even into the ankle or toes. A history of an immediate preceding trauma, a fall, a blow, or an incident of heavy lifting need not be elicited. In fact, the immediate relationship of stress and the onset of pain is infrequent. The strain or repeated stresses have frequently occurred prior to the acute onset and have set the stage for the ultimate herniation. By *setting the stage* is meant the weakening of the annulus fibrosus which diminishes the elastic recoil against a stress. A minimal stress applied on the disc that is contained within a weakened defective annulus may cause the nuclear material to herniate.

The onset of sciatica ordinarily is abrupt. Pain most frequently begins as a low back pain, which usually is situated in the region of the lumbosacral spine but according to the patient's complaint it may run

146

across the whole low back or may restrict itself to one side of the lower region of back. As a rule, the pain initiates a sufficient spasm that immobilizes trunk function. As a result, the patient is unable to bend or to arise to a full erect position without evoking some degree of discomfort. Any movement of the trunk initiates spasm and pain.

In a large percentage of patients, pain is felt in the lower area of the back and simultaneously along the leg. Pain may be felt as a sensation of aching or "spasm" in the anterior upper thigh area. The spine splints into an antalgic posture (flattening of the lordosis), movement becomes restricted, and usually an acute functional scoliosis develops.

Sciatic pain, usually considered a pressure neuritis, is a pain due to nerve irritation that is referred down the leg. The patient's description actually points out to the examiner the specific nerve root and essentially the extent to which the nerve is being irritated. The usual distribution of this pain referral involves the buttocks, the posterior thigh, the calf, the heel, and the toes.

The pain of peripheral neuropathy, commonly called *sciatica,* has been attributed to numerous causative factors. Sciatica was originally considered to be due to spasm of the hamstring muscles acting in a "protective" manner.[4,5] It was later considered to be a traction neuropathy when the nerve root was observed to move in the intervertebral foramen during the straight-leg raising test.[6]

Recent studies seem to indicate an ischemia as the major cause, yet this does not answer the immediate onset of pain immediately following nerve compression. Root irritation due to compression by the disc is being questioned when 88.8 percent of the patients with a positive Laségue test had subsequent negative surgical exploration.[7]

Mere contact with an *inflamed* root is an adequate stimulus for pain of a sciatic distribution, regardless of what has caused the irritation or compression.[8] Pain radiating further down the leg implicates a greater area of nerve contact.

Mechanism

The mechanism by which disc herniation occurs and the process by which it causes the symptoms and manifests diagnostic signs can now be described in its chronological sequence. The immediate pain that follows the herniation of the lumbar disc *in the back* is due to muscle spasm, concomitant facet approximation with an acute synovitis, and in part painful irritation of the recurrent nerve of Luschka (Fig. 103).

In the leg, the site to which pain is referred is the dermatome area of a specific nerve root (Fig. 104). The particular nerve root which is irritated is dependent upon the level of intervertebral disc at which the nerve root emerges. How far the pain or numbness will run down the

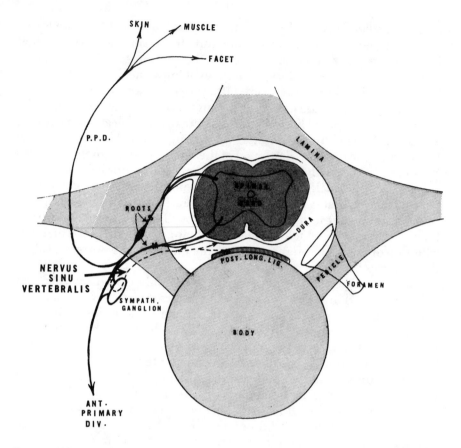

SKIN

MUSCLE

FACET

P.P.D.

LAMINA

SPINAL CORD

ROOTS

DURA

NERVUS
SINU
VERTEBRALIS

POST. LONG. LIG.

PEDICLE

FORAMEN

SYMPATH.
GANGLION

BODY

ANT.
PRIMARY
DIV.

FIGURE 103. Sinu vertebralis nerve. The recurrent nerve of Luschka is considered to convey sensory fibers to the posterior longitudinal ligament, the dura, and reaching to the outer border of the annulus.

length of the patient's leg is dependent on the extent of the pressure on the nerve at the intervertebral foramen. After the patient indicates in his case history all the above-mentioned factors, the physical examination then objectively verifies the site and magnitude of the disc herniation.

A patient's history of the onset of disc herniation does not always present a precise *cause and effect* story. In an attempt to elicit a history of severe stress immediately followed by low back pain, with or without sciatica, the examiner is likely to find himself frequently uninformed or even misinformed. The stress immediately preceding the onset of pain may be described as mild, and the history of *any* stress often is actually unobtainable. A past history of frequent, mild, an occasional severe, or intermittent mild and severe attacks of low back pain often can be

148

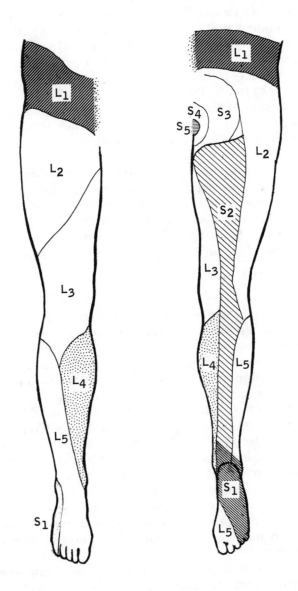

FIGURE 104. Sensory dermatome area map. The areas mapped out are the areas of hypalgesia to pin-scratch testing. Because of patient variation, the areas at best are general and overlapping.

drawn from the patient. Which of these previous episodes set the stage for the present acute and severe incident still remains a mystery.

Each episode of trauma has apparently set the stage for ultimate extrusion of the nucleus into the annular tears. Now a minor stress can "tip the scales." Occasionally the precipitating episode is severe and pain follows immediately. Most patients, however, recall only a minor strain followed by symptoms of low back pain and nerve root irritation. A sequence of mild strains initiating severe symptoms leads to the frequent controversy of *cause and effect* in medicolegal decisions and in dispositions of industrial injury claims.

In the evolution of the mechanism of disc herniation, the various factors elicited in the history can be correlated. Repeated minor traumata, with no sciatic radiation but with resultant low back pains, may well have been the episodes that gradually weakened the annulus. These repeated strains may be a series of strains from the lifting of heavy objects or may be acute facet impingements from minor physical activities. They may have been innocuous lifting or bending incidents but there was a mild structural back defect in the person who performed them. All of these have the ability to set the stage for ultimate disc herniation producing subjective and objective signs and symptoms.

Diagnosis

The onset of the pain may be related to the back alone or exclusively to symptoms in the leg. Both, however, may occur simultaneously. The initial symptoms may be described as sharp, dull, continuous, or intermittent. Numbness of the leg may precede or accompany the symptom of pain. Relationship to activities or positions at which symptoms appear may vary, and various positions or activities may relieve the symptoms or vary the character and extent of the site of the symptoms. All of these variations have a mechanical and pathophysiologic explanation. Careful interpretation of the symptoms does not lead merely to accurate diagnosis but also informs the examiner of the extent of herniation, the exact vertebral level of the herniation, and postulates the course of the disease and its prognosis (Table 1).

The examination, which is relatively simple and can proceed rapidly, merely verifies the impression created by the history. The necessity of many laboratory tests may be eliminated by careful systematic history and examination.

Sciatic pain is rare in an acute strain with facet impingement. Although pressure from the strain is exerted on the disc, the symptoms actually result from an acute synovitis of the compressed facets or from overstretched ligaments. If sciatic pain is present, the complaint is rarely substantiated by *objective* findings of nerve irritation. Most

150

TABLE 1. Clinical Features for Differential Diagnosis of Back Pain*

	Trauma		
	Joint	Muscle	Disc Prolapse
Onset	Sudden During movement With snap or lock	Sudden With lifting With tearing feeling	Sudden With stressful move With lock
Effect of rest	Relieving	Stiffening	Relieving, especially with partial flexion
Effect of activity	Aggravating	Aggravating	Aggravating
Location	Over junction or sacroiliac joint	Over muscle	Over junction
Architectural changes	Segmental alteration of normal curve Curve convex on side of pain Iliac crest raised on side of pain	No change in spinal curve — —	Segmental alteration of normal curve Curve concave on side of pain Iliac crest lower on side of pain
Mobility	Localized loss Recovery straight	Less well localized Recovery tortuous or straight	Localized loss Recovery straight
Percussion	Short sharp pain	—	Short sharp pain, often with radiation
Obvious physical signs	One joint One level Unilateral Pain may be referred No neurologic signs	No joint No area Unilateral Pain in muscle No neurologic signs	One junction Same level joint Bilateral Radiating pain Mixed neurologic signs
General observations	Patient lies still No signs of systemic disease No fever	Patient varies position No signs of systemic disease No fever	Patient lies still No signs of systemic disease No fever
X-ray findings	Negative	Negative	Negative except with special techniques
Laboratory findings	Negative	Negative	Negative except CSF protein often increased

*Modified from Mennell, J.M.: Differential diagnosis of visceral from somatic back pain. J. Occup. Med. 8(9):477–480, 1966.

151

patients with this condition have relatively free trunk flexion but lack the ability to hyperextend or "arch the back" without causing pain. In trunk flexion the facets are separated or disengaged, whereas in extension they are further "jammed" together and the inflamed surfaces are compressed.

Pain and sensitivity in the motor points of the involved muscles, discussed previously, may indicate the specific level of root irritation but not necessarily implicate a disc herniation. The "absence" of neurologic deficit may merely mean that there is no *gross loss* of reflexes, muscle strength, or sensation, but subtle signs can be elicited if carefully sought. These imply skin sensitivity to "rolling" or vasomotor changes.[9,10] All these subtle signs must be absent before it can be claimed that no neurologic deficit is present.

In the examination of the patient with low back pain suspected of being caused by a mechanical abnormality, the standing posture has diagnostic characteristics. The usual physiologic lordosis becomes straightened. The lumbar spine becomes "straight" or kyphotic (Fig. 105). This is manifested clinically and can be noted on routine x-rays of the lumbosacral spine. Having the patient attempt to flex forward reveals no movement of the lumbar spine with the patient bending at the hips and the lumbar spine remains rigid.

The "spasm" that restricts lumbar movement is a protective mechanism to prevent elongation of the spinal canal which elongates the posterior longitudinal ligament and causes migration of the nerve roots and their dura. If there is a protrusion of the intervertebral disc, the involved nerve root is tethered across this protrusion.[11]

Viewing the patient attempting to laterally flex, to the right then the left, reveals limited restriction at one segment, but this can be noted only at the upper lumbar vertebrae as it is unusual to detect any movement normally below the fourth lumbar vertebra.

A functional scoliosis is often present in lumbar disc herniation. Lateral deviation of the spine is often to the side *away* from the involvement of the nerve root, but this is not a constant or a diagnostic factor. Scoliosis is considered to be a reflex splinting of the lumbar spine (Fig. 106).

The *straight-leg raising test* is a delicate and accurate neurologic test. The straight-leg raising test (from this point to be designated the *SLR*) is currently used interchangeably with the terms *positive* or *negative* Laségue sign. The SLR, when done carefully, and properly interpreted, is one of the few tests that offer objective diagnostic signs.

The SLR is not in actuality the Laségue sign. In the SLR, the leg is flexed at the hip with the knee held in full extension. The ankle, during the exercise, remains in a relaxed position. Forst was the first to describe this test. The test described by Laségue was that of flexion of the

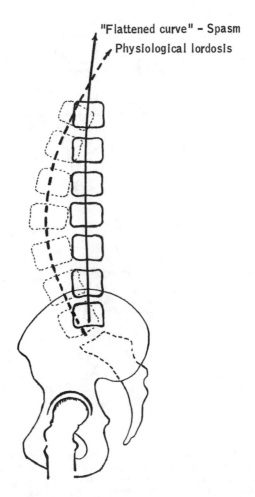

"Flattened curve" – Spasm

Physiological lordosis

FIGURE 105. Lumbar spasm with resultant "flattening." The spasm resulting from nerve root irritation causes a protective spasm. This spasm, rather than increasing the lordosis, results in straightening the lumbar curve. Further forward flexion of the lumbar curve is prevented by this spasm.

hip to 90 degrees, followed by extension of the lower leg in line with the thigh. The term *Laségue* now has clinical acceptance as being synonymous with SLR. If, however, either test is interpreted correctly, the designation employed is of no importance.

During SLR the first 15 to 30 degrees of elevation causes no movement of the nerve roots at the foraminal level. But when the leg has reached an angle of 30 degrees, there is traction on the sciatic nerve followed by a downward movement of the roots in their foramina. The greatest degree of movement occurs in the L_5 root, some slight movement at L_4, and essentially no movement at L_2 or L_3. The greatest

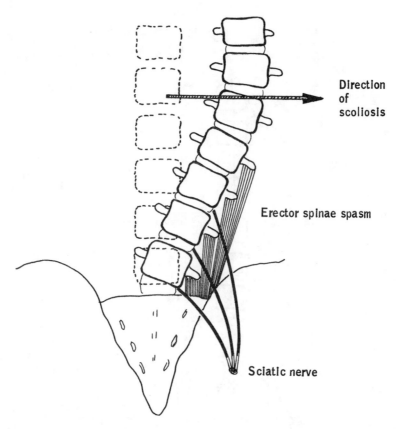

Direction
of
scoliosis

Erector spinae spasm

Sciatic nerve

FIGURE 106. Mechanism of acute protective scoliosis. Irritation of the nerve root at its emergence through the intervertebral foramen causes reflex spasm, usually on the same side as the site of irritation. By its segmental distribution, only a small portion of the paraspinous muscles is involved, and thus a segmental lateral curve of the spine results.

distance of any root movement, a distance of 2 to 5 mm, occurs when the SLR has brought the leg to an angle of 60 to 80 degrees.[12,13]

The clinical interpretation urged by these facts is that owing to the greatest downward movement occurring at the L_5 level, a disc herniation at this level will have a strongly felt positive reaction from the SLR. As there is a decreasing amount of reaction at the higher nerve root levels, a disc herniation at the level of L_3 or even L_4 may not produce a positive SLR. A positive SLR is of greatest value in helping to locate a disc herniation at the L_5-S_1 and L_{4-5} level, but its absence does not argue against a disc herniation existing at a higher interspace.

In the young there are few fibrous adhesions that attach the nerve roots to the foraminae, thus the nerve roots have greater movement. As a person ages, the nerve roots become more adherent and accordingly there is less downward movement. The nerves thus become more tense in their attempt to assume a straight course,[14] and pressure over bony prominences increases.

Lessening of the lumbar lordosis (at necropsy) was found to cause a slight separation of the pedicles of the foramen, thus opening the foramen. This allowed the roots to run a more direct (straight, rather than curved) course and thus be slackened (see Fig. 91). This may explain the "natural" assumption of the antalgic spine in acute sciatica (see Fig. 105).

Excessive lordosis also increases the bulging posteriorly of the disc as well as the bunching of the ligamentum flavum. This decreases in the slightly flexed lumbar spine. Also, in mid-flexed posture, the spinal canal length is optimal to minimize traction upon the nerve roots.

After reaching the limit of SLR, as determined by pain or discomfort, having the patient flex his neck (chin to chest) will cause or aggravate the pain down the nerve root distribution. This can be considered a confirmatory sign to the Laségue test.

Nuchal flexion elongates the dural sac cranially as the straight-leg raise elongates the dural sac distally. Maximal elongation of the dura is probably performed by total trunk flexion which, in the standing position, causes hip flexion (straight leg raising). If this is followed by forced neck flexion, signs of dural traction will be revealed.

Normally the dural sleeve of the nerve roots is slack. In full flexion the dura elongates. In straight-leg raising (SLR), the dura is pulled against the ligament that attaches the nerve root to the foramen, and the dura becomes taut. If there has been no inflammation or trauma to the nerve, no symptoms result. If there is a disc herniation that presses upon the nerve root, the root dura is pulled cephalad, causing distal tautness (Fig. 107). SLR increases the tautness, as does the nuchal flexion which draws the dura cephalad.

The constriction of the dural sleeve follows the laws of tensile force expended upon a flexible tube in which the tensile force decreases the circumference of the tube for a distance down the tube, from the site of the force, for a distance three times that of the diameter (Fig. 108).

This explains the nerve constriction with resultant ischemia and the effect of the disc protrusion, SLR, and nuchal flexion. It also explains that compression from the disc is not, by itself, the total explanation of ischemia with resultant pain and dysfunction.

A different manner of performing the SLR test that has proved of sufficient value to merit discussion has been that of performing the test while the patient is sitting. With legs dangling, the patient is seated on the edge of the table, and faces the examiner. The test then is merely performed by extending the patient's legs below the knee one at a time. The examiner should note the results objectively and subjectively.

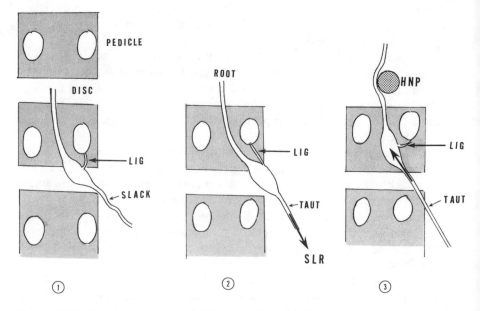

FIGURE 107. Nerve root traction. 1. The normal root with a slack ligament and full flexibility. 2. With straight-leg raising, the nerve root dura becomes taut. 3. With a herniated disc pressing upon the nerve root, the root is pulled cephalad and increases the tautness distally.

This apparently trivial modification of the test described by Lasègue in respect to the supine position has several benefits. In the supine position, raising a straight leg manually can be difficult because the patient may squirm and shift his pelvis, thus making the leg abduct and rotate. Furthermore the apprehension of the patient to ward off anticipated pain may cause SLR to render positive reaction far sooner than the objective facts warrant. In the supine position the back may be in a flexed or an extended position which may influence the test and cause difficulty in its proper interpretation.

In the sitting position, however, the patient faces the examiner and feels more secure and at ease. The examiner is able to determine immediately the slightest attempt on the part of the patient to withdraw by leaning back from the pain induced by the straight-leg raising. Indication that the pain level has been reached may be given by the facial grimace of the patient or by his "general bracing" against further leg elevation. Moreover, it is no easier to note and record the precise degree of elevation (e.g., 45°, 65°, etc.) from the test taken in the supine position. Neither method can be said to be more accurate or significant than the other.

The results of the SLR test should be expressed in terms of *positive* or

156

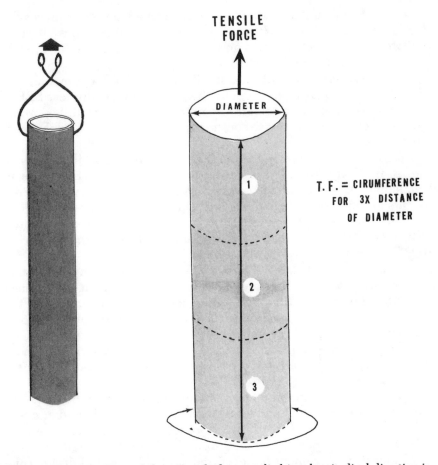

TENSILE
FORCE

DIAMETER

T. F. = CIRUMFERENCE
FOR 3X DISTANCE
OF DIAMETER

FIGURE 108. Saint-Venant's law. Tensile force applied in a longitudinal direction is distributed uniformly around the circumference for a distance equal to three times the diameter of the tube. Tension thus applied to the nerve root dura is transmitted as a compression force for a distance of three times the diameter of the root, both cranially and caudally. This explains radicular pain caused by an HNP, SLR, and nuchal flexion.

negative. The test is essentially qualitative rather than quantitative. As a rule, to be termed positive the test is so unilaterally.

In patients suspected of falsifying or magnifying their symptoms, the SLR may be performed with the patient seated. The leg can be slowly elevated while the patient is simultaneously distracted by any guise of the examiner. If pain is elicited by SLR in this manner before the test can be considered "positive," ankle dorsiflexion and nuchal flexion should be performed for confirmation.

In nerve entrapment from L_3 and cephalad (L_2-L_1), the nerve roots do not migrate with straight leg raising; therefore the Laségue test is negative. By placing the patient in the prone position which places the hip in extension, flexion of the knee (bringing the knee to the buttocks) irritates the L_3-L_4 nerve roots and causes radiation down the anterior thigh: the femoral nerve distribution.

A "crossed sciatica" SLR is a significant test implying marked encroachment upon that nerve root. In the performance of this test, SLR of the "normal" leg causes referred pain down the opposite leg. Many surgeons consider this test to confirm the need for surgical exploration when positive.[15]

Traction on the nerve by SLR, trunk flexion, or nuchal flexion is *not* necessary to initiate pain. Pressure on the nerve alone can result in immediate pain of a *sharp* character. This pain is more severe when it occurs in a previously irritated nerve. The extent of the pressure over a specified area, not the duration or the intensity of pressure, determines how far down the sciatic nerve dermatome distribution the pain is felt by the patient.[16]

When the patient states "the pain goes so far down my leg," he is apparently describing how much of a herniated fragment is in contact with the nerve root. When the patient specifies a particular area of the lower extremity, he is specifying the root level that supplies that dermatomal or myotomal region (Fig. 109).

When numbness replaces pain as a symptom, it may indicate more massive and more prolonged pressure upon the nerve root. Weakness implies even greater pressure.

A central disc herniation can present a diagnostic problem. By its central herniation the fragment is in direct contact with neither nerve root, and thus pain or paresthesia is not felt in either lower extremity. Merely low back pain is felt, and trunk flexion is restricted.

If a facet impingement has occurred, and not a central disc herniation, functional scoliosis may be present. Limited trunk flexibility may be noted, but in this condition there is usually more pain on trunk hyperextension than on flexion. Time with periodic observation may be necessary to designate precisely the true etiology of the pain.

Persistence of scoliosis with limitation of trunk flexion and persistence of pain upon straight-leg raising unilaterally or bilaterally in spite of prolonged conservative treatment favor the diagnosis of central disc herniation rather than facet impingement.

In acute "facet synovitis" the articulations disengage, scoliosis subsides, and the straight-leg raising permits greater elevation with less pain. Trunk flexion increases with greater reversal of the lordosis, and even painless hyperextension is possible. Hyperextension may remain painful and limited.

Persistence of scoliosis with or without pain and with limited trunk lateral flexion can imply a facet joint minor dysfunction with mechani-

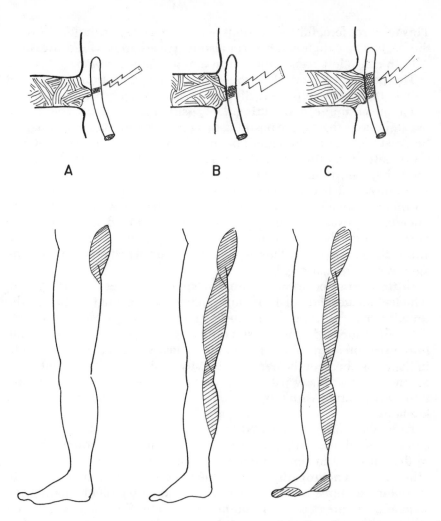

FIGURE 109. Subjective area of referred pain: correlation with area of nerve contact. *A.* A slight degree of nerve contact will cause the patient to claim pain that is referred to the buttocks region. *B.* Pain claimed to radiate down the posterior thigh, with or without buttocks pain, implies a greater degree of nerve contact. *C.* Pain referred to the foot region implies a larger area of nerve contact and also gives an indication of the root spinal level. The amount of pressure is not so important as is the extent of the nerve contact at the foraminal level.

cal "locking." Lateral flexion exercises or manipulation may be suggested (see Chapter 4).

The presence of pain "running down" the leg, elicited by coughing or sneezing, is strongly suggestive of disc herniation but is *not conclusive.* To accomplish its primary purpose, a cough must initiate intrapleural and intra-abdominal pressure by means of a Valsalva manuever.

This requires forceful contractions of many muscles, including those of the back. The cough mechanism also increases spinal fluid pressure. All can cause low back pain, but in a nonspecific manner.

The patient's history describes causation, aggravation, or relief of pain in its relationship to gravity. A patient may get relief from becoming prone or supine, or by sitting. The position of the back, either flexed or extended in the supine position, that causes or relieves the pain must be noted. Sitting is often more painful than standing, which relates to the greater intradiscal pressure from this position[17] or to the flexed lumbar spine in the seated position.

Studies of the hydrodynamics of the lumbar disc have cast some light on this phenomenon. The intradiscal pressure—pressure within the nucleus pulposus and thus within the intervertebral disc—is less by 30 percent in the lying than in the standing position and is greater in sitting than in standing. This explains the value of bed rest as well as the aggravation from sitting.[18]

In the sitting position the lumbar spine becomes forward-flexed, which elongates the canal and thus can impose cephalad traction on the dura.[19,20] This position can intensify the radicular pain.

Bending forward from the standing or sitting position increases the intradiscal pressure. This is even more aggravated if a weight is held in the arms ahead of the center of gravity. This accounts undoubtedly for the fact that many patients develop low back and radicular pain from this position which is so common in industry and in household kitchens.

Radicular pain or an irritated sciatic nerve may persist after removal of a herniated disc, after regression of disc irritation ("natural" history of disc disease) in sciatic neuropathy *without* disc herniation, or in other forms of neuropathy. This is due to persistence of hyperirritability of lumbar nerve roots which will respond with radicular pain when touched, compressed, or placed under traction. This may account for the benefit of treating sciatica with steroids and the occurrence of sciatica with a "negative" myelogram or after "successful" surgery.

Neurologic Examination and Interpretation

The specific nerve root involvement can be clinically determined but does not indicate the specific lumbar disc. This becomes evident in reviewing the anatomical course of the nerve roots in their passage distally past the disc spaces (Fig. 110).

The specific nerve root(s) can be determined by a careful neurologic examination that includes testing deep tendon reflexes, sensory "mapping" examinations, and a test of each muscle innervated by the specific myotomes (Fig. 111 and Table 2).

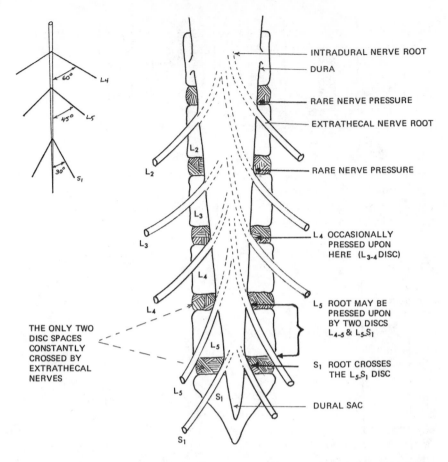

INTRADURAL NERVE ROOT

DURA

RARE NERVE PRESSURE

EXTRATHECAL NERVE ROOT

RARE NERVE PRESSURE

L₄ OCCASIONALLY PRESSED UPON HERE (L₃₋₄ DISC)

L₅ ROOT MAY BE PRESSED UPON BY TWO DISCS L₄₋₅ & L₅S₁

S₁ ROOT CROSSES THE L₅S₁ DISC

DURAL SAC

THE ONLY TWO DISC SPACES CONSTANTLY CROSSED BY EXTRATHECAL NERVES

FIGURE 110. Relationship of specific nerve root to corresponding intervertebral disc.

Pain down the lower extremity suggests lumbosacral caudal root irritation. When related to lumbar flexion, a positive SLR (Laségue) heightens the probability of involvement of lower roots (L₄₋₅-S₁), as involvement higher up (L₁₋₂₋₃) usually does not cause a positive Laségue (SLR) test. The patient's subjective localization of the pain or numbness gives a good indication of the dermatome which then can be confirmed by careful examination.

It is redundant to specify that the neurologic examination should include upper motor neuron testing for hyperactive reflexes, Babinski, clonus, etc. Lesions involving the cauda equina could not cause upper motor neuron signs.

Muscle testing is a reliable method to specify a myotome (motor root). The gastroc soleus (S₁) is difficult to test manually as it is a powerful

TABLE 2. Schematic Dermatome and Myotome Level of Nerve Root Impingement

Nerve Root	Inter-vertebral Space	Subjective Pain Radiation	Sensory Area	Bladder Bowel Dysfunction*	SLR†	Ankle Jerk‡	Knee Jerk‡	Motor Dysfunction (Myotome)§
L₃	L₂-L₃	Back to buttocks to posterior thigh to anterior knee region	Hypalgesia in knee region	+/-	Usually -	+	+	Quadriceps weakness
L₄	L₃-L₄	Back to buttocks to posterior thigh to inner calf region	Hypalgesia inner aspect of lower leg	+/-	Usually - May be +	+	-	Quadriceps and possible anticus weakness
L₅	L₄-L₅	Back to buttocks to dorsum of foot and big toe	Hypalgesia in dorsum foot and big toe	+/-	++	+	+	Weakness of anterior tibialis, big toe extensor, gluteus medius
S₁	L₅-S₁	Back to buttocks to sole of foot and heel	Hypalgesia in heel or lateral foot	+/-	+++	-	+	Weakness of gastrocnemius, hamstring, gluteus maximus

*Bladder and bowel dysfunction can occur at any level.
†Related to extent of nerve root movement at each level.
‡Ankle jerk is absent only at L₅-S₁; knee jerk at L₃-L₄.
§Only the more obvious and functional muscles are listed.

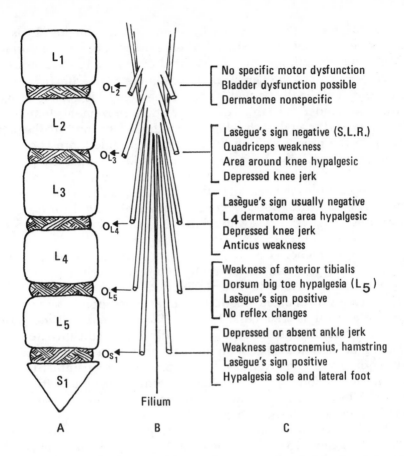

FIGURE 111. Clinical localization of dermatome-myotome level of disc herniation. *A*. Lateral view of the spine showing the nerve root relationship to the intervertebral disc (e.g., S_1 nerve root at level of disc between vertebra L_5 and first sacral vertebra S_1). *B*. Indication of the level at which the cord becomes the cauda equina (L_1). Below this level any nerve injury is equivalent to a peripheral nerve injury. *C*. The clinical manifestations of the various nerve roots as found on neurologic examination.

muscle that is difficult to resist and to grade unless it is markedly paralyzed. With the patient upright, rising upon the toes, one foot at a time, will utilize the patient's body weight for resistance.

Having the patient perform many elevations "up on the toes" will reveal fatigue of the involved S_1 nerve root. This is a subtle test that reveals S_1 root involvement often when one elevation will not reveal significant weakness.

The anterior tibialis (L_5) ankle dorsiflexor can be grossly tested by having patients walk on their heels. A more precise evaluation of the anterior tibialis can be performed by manually resisting ankle dorsiflexion for strength and repeatedly for endurance.

Testing the big toe extensor (extensor hallucis longus) L_5 is very sensitive and may be "positive" when grosser muscles test normally. Again the strength loss may be verified by testing for endurance.

The strength of the hamstring group in their knee flexing action is best tested while the patient is seated and bends his knee to bring his lower leg under the table. In this position, movement done against resistance is better than the standard method of testing with the patient lying in the prone position. In the prone attitude there is a marked tendency to arch the back which is not evident when the patient is sitting. Avoidance of too much reclining, turning, sitting, and rolling over is desirable for a patient with a low back pain or herniated lumbar disc. The hamstring muscle group is innervated by S_1 primarily and confirms weakness already noted in the gastrocnemius-soleus (S_1) and the big toe extensor (S_1).

To test the higher nerve roots (L_3-L_4) the strength of the quadriceps femoris group is tested. This muscle group extends the leg at the knee. As the quadriceps muscle is very powerful, it may be necessary to have the person do repeated one-legged deep knee bends to determine fatigue as well as weakness. In more marked weakness the patient, while in the sitting position, may be unable to maintain full extension of the leg at the knee against slight manual pressure. The quadriceps strength test may be invalidated in the presence of a painful SLR when the testing is done with the patient seated. If sciatic neuritis or tight hamstrings is suspected of restricting knee extension, the quadriceps may be tested with the patient supine.

It is seriously recommended that the patient be examined in the *upright* position when the strength of the antigravity muscle is tested. The present-day manner of examining the patient draped and lying on an examining table leaves many significant factors unnoticed. Even the examination with the patient in a sitting position is inadequate for thorough evaluation. Where this applies in posture and kinetic function evaluation, so in the same way it must be employed in muscle testing. It is inconceivable that in an attempt to determine deviation from normal, one should not be examined in his normal upright stance and in his antigravity functions.

Further phases of the neurologic examination can also be performed with the patient seated. After the completion of the SLR testing, examination of the deep tendon jerks is made. The reflexes are evaluated with reference to their presence, and comparison is made of relation of one side to the other. The deep tendon reflexes reflect peripheral nerve integrity and therefore are a test of lower motor neuron function. In essence the reflexes are tested to determine the spinal segmental level of any suspected nerve root compression. Depression of one side as compared to the other is of significance because pressure on the nerve

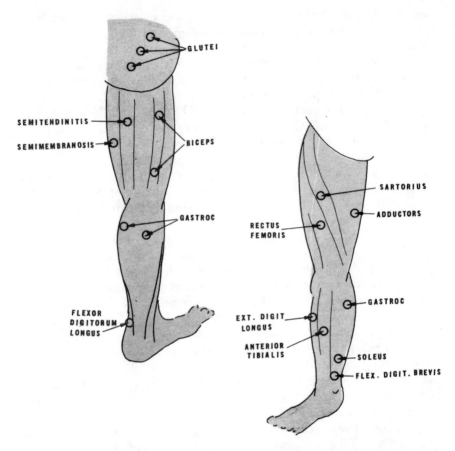

FIGURE 112. Tender motor points at sites of myoneural junction. On deep pressure these sites of tenderness conform to the muscles innervated by the root at a specific intervertebral space.

root will result in depression of the reflex. Significant pressure on a nerve root may result in total loss of a deep tendon reflex.

The ankle jerk (AJ) is dependent on an intact S_1 motor root. A depressed knee jerk (KJ) implicates pressure on the L_4 root. Active symmetrical knee and ankle jerks are expected when there is nerve root compression at L_5 as this nerve root does not innervate a tendon reflex. Pressure on the nerve root at this level (L_5) requires sensory and motor testing to establish the diagnosis.

Absence of *bilateral* deep tendon reflexes at one level is possible in a central disc herniation at a segmental level when both left and right nerve roots are encroached upon. Although neither motor nor sensory deficit may exist with areflexia, some nerve impairment exists, and other signs of lumbar-disc herniation should exist, such as bilateral positive SLR reactions, lumbar spine spasm, scoliosis, and subjective unilateral or bilateral sciatica.

The sensory examination follows in the neurologic appraisal. A pin is "run down" (that is, applied with a light scratching maneuver rather than by "sticking") the inner side of each leg into the foot area, then down the lateral aspect of the legs, the bilateral heel areas, lateral aspects of the foot, and the dorsum of the big toes. This method aids the patient to ascertain differences more easily as the dermatome maps overlap and the scratch does not demand a distinct border of any area. Suffice to say that the *difference* of sensation of the right compared to left is the objective of the test—not merely the ability of the patient "to feel the pin scratch." Nerve root compression results in impaired sensation of the specific dermatome area, varying from hypalgesia to complete anaesthesia. Hyperesthesia on the basis of nerve irritation is rarely found in nerve root involvement due to disc protrusion, although it is theoretically possible to have irritation hyperesthesia.

There are many patients who have low back pain after a "strain" and demonstrate no localizing physical findings in the usual standard physical examination or from confirmatory tests. These patients are considered to be suffering from "low back sprain,"[24] and when their symptoms persist, they are frequently accused of having psychosocial or monetary gain motivation.

If these patients are specifically examined, they may demonstrate tenderness at the motor points of the muscles innervated by the roots emerging from that specific vertebral segment[25] (Fig. 112). These tender motor points were discovered when performing electromyographic examinations of the muscles innervated by the myotome roots emerging from a specific functional unit. The EMG findings were of increased insertional potential, prolongation of the duration of motor unit potential, and partial interference potential during maximal voluntary effort.[26] The motor points are fixed anatomical sites with little variation from person to person (Table 3). *These points are found to be tender in patients who simultaneously complain of low back pain.* The tender motor points can be palpated by firm finger pressure with significant firmness to compress the motor end-plate zone against the underlying bone.

The motor points of the posterior primary division to the paravertebral muscles are situated approximately 2.5 cm (1.0 inch) from the midline at the segmental level. These tender motor points are examined with the patient in the prone position, then the patient is examined in the supine position.

Tender motor points are occasionally found in normal asymptomatic individuals and in patients with significant disc degeneration. Often

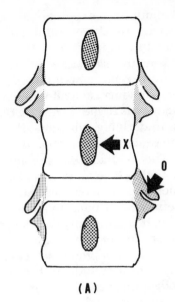

(A)

FIGURE 113. Examination to localize joint dysfunction. *A*. Lateral manual movement of posterior superior spine (X) localizes site of pathology. *B*. Pressure and deep paraspinous tissues over facets add localizing confirmation.

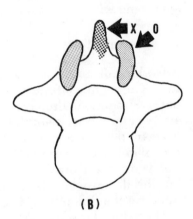

(B)

tender motor points are confused with conditions such as a trochanteric "bursitis," gluteal bursitis, or sciatic nerve tenderness in the sciatic notch area.

Finding these tender motor points may also coincide with the painful movement of the functional unit described by Maigne.[27] At the specifically involved segment, lateral pressure and movement of the posterior superior spine are painful. It is Maigne's concept that joint dysfunction causes both local and referred pain (Fig. 113). This is corroborated by finding localized deep tenderness over the facet joints at that same segment by deep digital pressure. Both points are similar in location and corroborate each other.

167

Many "trigger points" advocated by Travel and coworkers[28,29] may in fact be sensitive motor points. These points also conform to acupuncture points.[30,31]

Sensitive skin depicted by the "rolling" examination technique can certainly be a manifestation of this neurophysiologic condition. Trophedema is an alteration of skin elasticity and its underlying subcutaneous tissue. In testing the skin for this finding, a patch of skin and its underlying subcutaneous tissue are squeezed and rolled between the examiner's thumb and index finger.

The skin and the subcutaneous tissue are firmer, thickened, and sensitive. The same area of skin, when indented by a blunt instrument such as a wooden matchstick, leaves an indenture that is deep, well-defined, and persists longer than if this test is performed on normal skin. It is mandatory that the contralateral side be similarly examined to determine a difference with "positive" findings on the suspected side.

Before it is pronounced *negative,* a "complete neurologic examination" must include all the usual techniques of reflex, motor, sensory, and subtle signs. Then and only then, with the history and a thorough musculoskeletal examination, can the patient suffering from a low back syndrome with or without radiculitis be properly diagnosed.

Confirmatory Tests

A working diagnosis is reached by the history and physical examination. There are confirmatory x-ray evidence and laboratory tests that deserve mention, although their thorough discussion and evaluation are beyond the scope of this presentation. The doctor should at least have an idea when to request such tests and how much can be gained from them. The interpretation of the specific tests, such as x-ray, electromyogram, and myelogram, is a function of the specialist in that field, but the doctor who has requested the report should be qualified to interpret the findings reported.

The value of confirmatory tests is limited but is specific. No individual test of its own is completely diagnostic. As in any field of medicine, laboratory tests should be considered as supplementary and confirmatory to the history and physical examination. Some of these tests will not be necessary, and it is the decision of the doctor to accept or reject certain tests. The doctor should certainly be able to explain their value to the patient as well as intelligently to discuss their results with the consultant.

X-ray studies by routine films are of surprisingly little value in the diagnosis of herniated lumbar discs. Finding "normal disc spaces" does not exclude the presence of disc herniation. X-rays do not in themselves localize the level of disc herniation causing clinical

168

TABLE 3. Relationship of Specific Roots, Muscles, and Peripheral Nerves

Root	Muscle	Peripheral Nerve
L_2	Sartorius (L_{2-3})	Femoral
	Pectineus (L_{2-3})	Obturator
	Adductor longus (L_{2-3})	Obturator
L_3	Quadriceps femoris (L_{2-3-4})	Femoral
L_4	Quadriceps femoris (L_{2-3-4})	Femoral
	Tensor fascia lata (L_{4-5})	Superior gluteal
	Tibialis anterior (L_{4-5})	Peroneal
L_5	Gluteus medius (L_{4-5} S_1)	Superior gluteal
	Semi-membranosis (L_{4-5} S_1)	Sciatic
	Semi-tendinosis (L_{4-5} S_1)	Sciatic
	Extensor hallucis longis (L_{4-5} S_1)	Deep peroneal
S_1	Gluteus maximus (L_{4-5} S_{1-2})	Inferior gluteal
	Biceps femoris—short head (L_5 S_{1-2})	Sciatic
	Semi-tendinosis (L_{4-5} S_1)	Sciatic
	Medial gastrocnemius (S_{1-2})	Tibial
	Soleus (S_{1-2})	Tibial
S_2	Biceps femoris—long head (S_{1-2})	Sciatic
	Lateral gastrocnemius (S_{1-2})	Tibial
	Soleus (S_{1-2})	Tibial

symptoms. Radiologic evidence of a "narrow disc space" merely indicates that the disc material has been extruded or is to some degree degenerated. When the intradiscal pressure that normally maintains separation of the vertebrae permits a narrowing of the intervertebral disc space, it is obviously deficient and this deficiency implies the presence of rupture or degeneration, but the x-ray will not differentiate these two entities.

Myelography, currently a pantopaque study, is essentially of value to localize the exact site of disc herniation or to eliminate the possibility of other pathology causing pain or dysfunction. It is used also to determine the presence of more than one disc herniation.[32,33] Merely to confirm that there is a disc protrusion as the cause of the clinical findings is less and less accepted.

Myelography is currently being used to diagnose spinal stenosis with patients who have pseudoclaudication. Patients who have nerve root lesions from intervertebral foramen stenosis may have normal or nondiagnostic myelograms.

Abnormal myelograms are found in persons who are symptom-free.[34] The literature currently has clearly stated that myelography as performed lately with dye has a high incidence of subsequent arachnoiditis. Indiscriminate use of myelography must be carefully avoided or minimized.[35]

Discography, the injection of dye into the disc nucleus, has equivocal advocacy. Its use to "specifically localize the offending disc" is claimed, but in many patients in their fourth or fifth decade, disc degeneration is commonplace and not necessarily causative of symptoms.

Electromyography (EMG) objectively confirms specific motor nerve root involvement and localizes that root. Involvement of the posterior primary division of a nerve root by testing the paraspinous area aids in localizing the specific root.

As demyelination does not occur for 19 to 21 days after nerve compression, early diagnostic use of electromyography has had limited value. Finding positive sharp waves can indicate nerve root irritation.

More recently electromyographic evaluations of H reflex, F waves, and ankle jerk latencies have indicated more sensitivity in localizing nerve root pathology and the level of involvement. Standardization of determination of these waves (i.e., H reflex, F wave and ankle jerk latency) and the ease of their being elicited at this time make their application less than universally accepted.[36,37]

SUMMARY

A carefully elicited history and a precise physical examination constitute the most specific manner of determining the diagnosis of lumbar disc pathology with all further tests being what they are intended to be—confirmatory.

REFERENCES

1. Farfan, H.F.: Mechanical Disorders of the Low Back. Lea & Febiger, Philadelphia, 1973, pp. 63-92.
2. Nachemson, A.: The influence of spinal movement on the lumbar intradiscal pressure and on the tensile stresses in the annulus fibrosis. Acta Orthop. Scand. 33:3, 1963.
3. Farfan, H.F., et al.: The effects of torsion on the lumbar intervertebral joints: the role of torsion in the production of disc degeneration. J. Bone Joint Surg. 52-A: 468, 1970.
4. Forst, J.J.: Contribution a l'étude dexique de la sciatique. Paris Thèse, no. 33, 1881.
5. Lasègue, C.: Considerations sur la sciatique. Arch. Gen. Med. 2:558, 1864.
6. Falconer, M.A., McGeorge, M., and Begg, A.C.: Observations on the cause and mechanism of symptom production in sciatica and low back pain. J. Neurol. Neurosurg. Psychiatry 11:13, 1948.
7. Spangfort, E.V.: The lumbar disc herniation. A computer-aided analysis of 2504 operations. Acta Orthop. Scand. (Suppl.) 142:1-95, 1972.
8. McNab, I.: Chemonucleolysis. Clin. Neurosurg. 20:183-192, 1973.
9. Gunn, C.C., and Milbrandt, W.E.: Early and subtle signs in low back sprain. Spine 3:267-281, 1978.
10. Gunn, C.C., and Milbrandt, W.E.: Tenderness at motor points: a diagnostic and prognostic aid for low back injury. J. Bone Joint Surg. 58-A(6):815-825, 1976.
11. Charnley, J.: Orthopaedic signs in the diagnosis of disc protrusion. Lancet 1:186-192, 1951.

12. Inman, V.T., and Saunders, J.B.: The clinico-anatomic aspect of the lumbosacral region. Radiology 38:669-687, 1942.
13. Edgar, M.A., and Park, W.M.: Induced pain patterns on positive straight-leg raising in lower lumbar disc protrusion. J. Bone Joint Surg. 56-B(4):658-667, 1974.
14. Goddard, M.D., and Reid, J.D.: Movements induced by straight-leg raising in the lumbosacral roots, nerves and plexus, and in the intrapelvic section of the sciatic nerve. J. Neurol. Neurosurg. Psychiatry 28:12-18, 1965.
15. Woodhall, B., and Hayes, G.J.: The well leg-raising test of Fajersztajn in the diagnosis of ruptured lumbar intervertebral disc. J. Bone Joint Surg. 32-A(4):786-792, 1950.
16. Inman, V.T., et al.: Referred pain from experimental irritative lesions, in Studies Relating to Pain in the Amputee, Series II, Issue 23, June 1952, pp. 49-78.
17. Nachemson, A., and Morris, J.M.: In vivo measurement of intradiscal pressure. J. Bone Joint Surg. 46-A(5):1077-1092, 1964.
18. Nachemson, A., and Elfstrom, G.: Intradiscal dynamic pressure measurements in lumbar discs. Scand. J. Rehab. Med. Suppl. 1, 1970.
19. Breig, A., and Marions, O.: Biomechanics of the lumbosacral nerve roots. Acta Radiol. 1:1141-1160, 1963.
20. Breig, A.: Effect of biomechanical phenomenon on function of central nervous system. Acta Neurochir. 26(4):345, 1972.
21. Lindahl, O.: Hyperalgesia of the lumbar nerve roots in sciatica. Acta Orthop. Scand. 37:367-374, 1966.
22. Smyth, M., and Wright, V.: Sciatica and the intervertebral disc. J. Bone Joint Surg. 40-A:1401-1418, 1955.
23. Lindahl, O., and Rexed, B.: Histological changes in spinal nerve roots of operated cases of sciatica. Acta Orthop. Scand. 20:215-225, 1951.
24. Gunn and Milbrandt, Early and subtle signs in low back sprain, op. cit.
25. Gunn and Milbrandt, Tenderness at motor points, op. cit.
26. Goodgold, J., and Eberstein, A.: Electrodiagnosis of Neuromuscular Diseases. Williams & Wilkins, Baltimore, 1972, pp. 6, 164.
27. Maigne, R.: Orthopedic Medicine: A New Approach to Vertebral Manipulation. Charles C Thomas, Springfield, Ill., 1972.
28. Travel, J., and Rinzler, S.H.: The myofascial genesis of pain. Postgrad. Med. 11:425-434, 1952.
29. Sola, A.E., and Williams, R.L.: Myofascial pain syndrome. Neurology 6:91-95, 1956.
30. Melzack, R., Stillwell, D.M., and Fox, E.J.: Trigger points and acupuncture points for pain correlation and implication. Pain 3(1):3-23, 1977.
31. Kao, F.F., and Kao, J.J.: Acupuncture Therapeutics. Eastern Press, New Haven, 1973.
32. Hakelius, A., and Hindmarsh, J.: The comparative reliability of preoperative diagnostic methods in lumbar disc surgery. Acta Orthop. Scand. 43:234-238, 1972.
33. Hakelius, A., and Hindmarsh, J.: The significance of neurological signs and myelographic findings in the diagnosis of lumbar root compression. Acta Orthop. Scand. 43:239-246, 1972.
34. McRae, B.L.: Asymptomatic intervertebral disc protrusions. Acta Radiol. 46:9-27, 1955.
35. Berg, A.: Clinical and myelographic studies of conservatively treated cases of lumbar intervertebral disc protrusion. Acta Chir. Scand. 104:124-129, 1953.
36. Kirwan, E.O., Leyshon, A., and Wynn Parry, C.B.: Root pain—diagnostic value of electrical studies (in press).
37. Goodgold and Eberstein, op. cit., pp. 245-263.

BIBLIOGRAPHY

Anderson, K.S., and Sneppen, O.: Comparative study of myelographic filling defects in root sheaths and operative findings in cases of suspected lumbar intervertebral disc herniation. Acta Orthop. Scand. 39:312-320, 1968.

Dilke, T.F.W., Burry, H.C., and Grahame, R.: Extradural corticosteroid injection in management of lumbar nerve root compression. Br. Med. 2:635-637, 1973.

Froning, E.C., and Frohman, B.: Motion of the lumbosacral spine after laminectomy and spine fusion. J. Bone Joint Surg. 50-A:897-918, 1968.

Geiger, L.E.: Fusion of vertebrae following resection of intervertebral disc. J. Neurosurg. 18(1):79-85, 1961.

Hause, F.B., and O'Connor, S.J.: Specific management for lumbar and sacral radiculitis. J.A.M.A. 166:1285-1290, 1958.

Herschensohn, H.L.: Disability of the back in industrial workers. Cal. Med. 92(1):31-34, 1960.

Hirsch, C.: Efficiency of surgery in low back disorders. J. Bone Joint Surg. 47-A(5):991-1004, 1965.

Kirgis, H.D., and Llewellyn, R.C.: Diagnosis and treatment of injuries to the lumbar intervertebral disc of industrial workers. J. South. Med. Assoc. 52(8):895-898, 1959.

Knutsson, B.: Electromyographic studies in the diagnosis of lumbar disc herniation. Acta Orthop. Scand. 28:290-299, 1959.

Krusen, E.M., and Ford, D.E.: Compensation factor in low back injuries. J.A.M.A. 166:10, 1958.

McNab, I., Cuthbert, H., and Godfred, C.M.: The incidence of denervation of the sacrospinalis muscles following spinal surgery. Spine 2(4):294-298, 1977.

Mathews, J.A.: Dynamic discography: a study of lumbar traction. Ann. Phys. Med. 9(7):275-279, 1968.

McKenzie, R.A.: Manual correction of sciatic scoliosis. N.Z. Med. J. 76:194-199, 1972.

Mensor, M.C.: Non-operative treatment, including manipulation, for lumbar intervertebral disc syndrome. J. Bone Joint Surg. 37-A(5):925-936, 1955.

Oudenhoven, R.C.: Paraspinal electromyography following facet rhizotomy. Spine 2(4):299-304, 1977.

Rosomoff, H.L., Gallo, A.E., Givens, F.T., and Kuehn, C.A.: Ceptometry as an adjunct to the evaluation of lumbar disc syndrome. J. Neurosurg. 33:67-74, 1970.

Rosomoff, H.L., et al.: Ceptometry in the evaluation of nerve root compression in the lumbar spine. Surg. Gynecol. Obstet. 117:263-270, 1963.

Scott, J.C.: Stress factor in the disc syndrome. J. Bone Joint Surg. 37-B(1):107-111, 1955.

See, D.H., and Kraft, G.H.: Electromyography in paraspinal muscles following surgery for root compression. Arch. Phys. Med. Rehab. 56:80-83, 1975.

Smith, L., and Brown, J.E.: Treatment of lumbar intervertebral disc lesions by direct injection of chymopapain. J. Bone Joint Surg. 49-B(3):502-519, 1967.

Smyth, M.J., and Wright, V.: Sciatica and the intervertebral disc. J. Bone Joint Surg. 40-A(6):1401-1418, 1958.

Taylor, T.K.F., and Weiner, M.: Great toe extension reflex in the diagnosis of lumbar disc disorder. Br. Med. J. 2:487-489, 1969.

Wiberg, G.: Back pain in relation to the nerve supply of the intervertebral disc. Acta Orthop. Scand. 19:211-221, 1949.

Wilson, J.C.: Low back pain and sciatica. J.A.M.A. 200(8):129-136, 1967.

Wiltse, L.L., Widell, E.H., and Yuan, H.A.: Chymopapain chemonucleolysis in lumbar disc disease. J.A.M.A. 231(5):474-479, 1975.

CHAPTER 7

Degenerative Disc Disease: Spondylosis

The integrity of the functional unit depends upon the adequacy of the intervertebral disc. In the anterior weight-bearing portion of the unit the hydrodynamic properties of the disc with its intradiscal pressure maintain the separation of adjacent vertebral bodies. This action elongates the spine, exerts tension upon the longitudinal ligaments, and simultaneously separates the zygoapophyseal joints posteriorly.

The foraminae are opened, the ligamentum flavum is kept taut, and the intertwined annular fibers are also placed under tension.

Degeneration of the disc apparently is an expected occurrence predictable in all humans. Puschel[1] claimed that by age 20, the disc has reached maximum development and degenerative changes appear. The sequence of degenerative changes revealed that degenerative changes in the posterior articulations followed changes within the disc.[2]

Changes in the intervertebral disc have been noted very early in life. At first concentric tears can be noted in the annular fibers, indicating a failure of the matrix to maintain contact of the annular fibers with each other[3] (Fig. 114).

Tears in the collagen fibers of the annulus appear early in the border between the nucleus and the cartilaginous plates and extend toward the center of the nucleus. This is contrary to the concept that rotatory trauma in later life causes rupture of the outer annular fibers.[4] However, both probably occur: the former as a natural evolution, the latter as superimposed trauma.

Gradually the outward intradiscal pressure causes radial tears to occur in the disc (see Fig. 114). Thus the intradiscal pressure decreases and the vertebral bodies are permitted to approximate (Fig. 115).

As the annular fibers rupture in the periphery of the discs, there is a connective tissue reaction in which blood vessels grow in from the long ligaments, gradually forming granular fibrous tissues. ♦

173

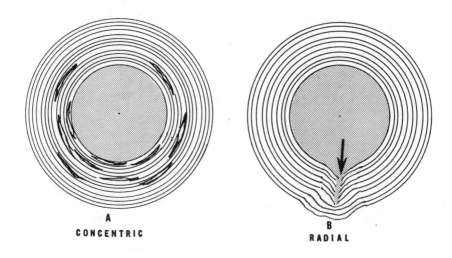

A
CONCENTRIC

B
RADIAL

FIGURE 114.   Annular changes in the degenerating disc. A reveals concentric tears in the annulus that are first noted at age 15. They originate near the nucleus and are at first discrete. As the patient ages, they are found in greater number in the outer margin and tend to merge into larger tears. B depicts radial tears. These too begin centrally and proceed outward. They are more numerous in the posterior portion of the disc. The pressure of the disc matrix pushes the torn fiber margins outward. When they reach the outer margin they "bulge" and deform the disc.

In the newborn child the vertebral column is straight and the intervertebral discs are wide and rectangular. As the child becomes weight-bearing and erect, the lordotic lumbar curve forms. The discs assume a wedge shape with posterior narrowing. The lumbosacral disc is even more wedge-shaped due to the lumbosacral angle. Degenerative changes are most prominent in the posterior lateral quadrants where the tissues capable of producing pain and disability are present.

Hereditary factors must predispose to premature disc degeneration. Some patients in their sixth or seventh decade are remarkably free of degenerative changes and are asymptomatic. Others as young as 20 may have significant degenerative changes. There does not appear to be any significant difference due to sex or occupation.[5]

The greatest degree of degeneration is noted at the lumbar (L_{4-5}) and the lumbosacral (L_5-S_1) intervertebral spaces (75 percent). This is possibly due to the greatest angulation of the intervertebral discs and the greatest proportion of lumbar movement at these two interspaces.

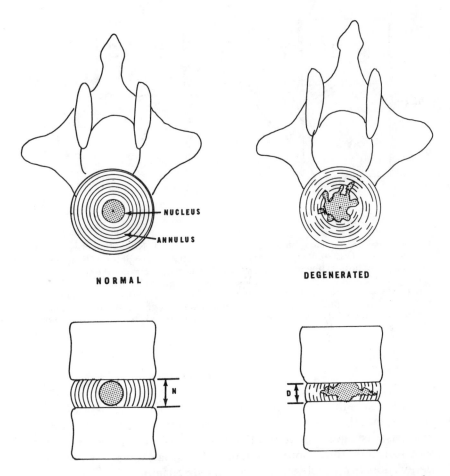

NUCLEUS

ANNULUS

NORMAL

DEGENERATED

N

D

FIGURE 115. Disc degeneration. *Left:* Normal disc with intact nucleus and annular fibers. The space is normal (N). *Right:* Degenerated disc with the nucleus outside its boundary and fragmented annular fibers and narrowed space (D).

As the anterior weight-bearing portion of the functional unit compresses due to disc dehydration, the posterior joints also approximate. These posterior joints undergo degenerative changes (e.g., synovial and capsular thickening, degeneration of articular cartilage, adhesions, osteochondral fractures, and even lose body formation). As there are fine sensory fibers that transmit pain and proprioception located in the capsules,[6] the posterior joints can now become symptomatic.

Gradual degenerative changes in all aspects of the functional unit lead to the condition termed *spondylosis* (Fig. 116).

175

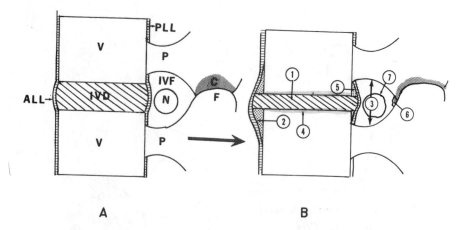

FIGURE 116. Sequence of degeneration: spondylosis. A. Normal functional unit: V = vertebral body; IVD = intervertebral disc; ALL = anterior longitudinal ligament; PLL = posterior longitudinal ligament; P = pedicle; N = nerve; IVF = intervertebral foramen; F = facet; and C = cartilage. B. Disc (1) degenerates; longitudinal ligament (2) slackens and pulls away from vertebral body; foramen (3) narrows; cartilaginous end plates (4) show sclerotic changes; posterior spurs or osteophytes (5) begin to form; degenerating cartilaginous changes (6) occur in facets; foraminal stenosis appears (7), leading to nerve root compression.

SPONDYLOSIS

The disease entity of *degenerative arthritis* of the spine is a sequela to intervertebral disc degeneration. Degenerative arthritis, hypertrophic arthritis, discogenic degenerative disease, osteoarthropathy, and spondylosis are morbidly and mechanically similar, toward which disc degeneration is undoubtedly a predisposing factor.

As the disc degenerates, the elastic fibers of the annulus decrease and are replaced by fibrous tissue. A loss of elasticity ensues, and flexibility of movement between two vertebrae is diminished. The intradiscal pressure that normally assists in keeping the vertebrae apart is decreased, and the vertebrae approximate. Shock-absorbing ability is decreased. The fibrous capsule and its ligaments become slack, and anterior-posterior shearing movement, normally not possible, can now occur.

Two pathologic conditions, capable of causing pain, result. The ligaments slacken when the vertebrae approximate, vertebral periosteal attachment of the ligaments weakens, and any pressure exerted on the ligament permits a dissection away from its periosteal attachment. Disc material usually confined within a taut ligamentous compartment can

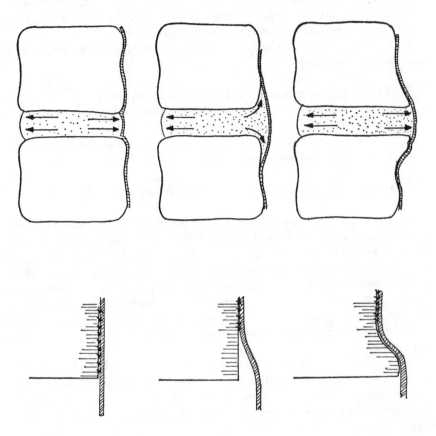

FIGURE 117. Mechanism of spondylosis. *Left:* The normal anterior portion of the functional unit with an intact disc, normal interspace, and a taut posterior longitudinal ligament that is totally adherent to the vertebral body periosteum. *Center:* Disc degeneration permits approximation of the two vertebrae, causing a slack in the posterior longitudinal ligament, and intradiscal pressure permits dissection between periosteum and ligament. *Right:* The extruded disc material becomes fibrous, then ultimately calcifies into what becomes a "spur."

now dissect the slack ligament from its previous site of attachment on the vertebrae (Fig. 117). Further extrusion of disc material is facilitated by the fragmentation of the annulus.

The material extruded decreases the quantity of disc tissue between the vertebrae and permits further vertebral approximation, further ligamentous laxity, more dissection of the ligamentous-periosteal attachment, and further protrusion of nuclear material: the process becomes a vicious circle. The extruded material, since it is a foreign body, evokes an irritation reaction. This irritation may be removed by fibrous

177

replacement followed by calcification. This calcified extruded tissue becomes the "arthritic spur" seen on x-ray film. Because of this the concept of spondylosis evolution appears feasible.

With these changes in the mobile portion of the lumbar spine, several conditions may result:

1. The usual symptoms of degenerative arthritis, such as early morning stiffness, constant aching, restricted range of motion, and limited duration of standing or sitting.
2. Nerve root entrapment due to intervertebral foramen narrowing.
3. Pseudoclaudication due to lumbar spine stenosis.

DISC DEGENERATION WITHOUT ROOT IRRITATION

The physical findings in chronic degenerative disc disease between acute exacerbations are not significant. Except for possible poor conditioning, poor posture, poor muscle tone, and limited flexibility, most patients with degenerative disc disease appear to be normal until an acute "attack" intervenes. Between attacks, a precise examination might reveal areas of deep tenderness in a specific paraspinous area or in motor point areas. Pressure on posterior superior spines in a lateral direction may elicit tenderness where acute pathology resulted (see Fig. 113).

Most often, even with normal flexion and good reversal of the lordosis, some discomfort or disruption of reextension can be noted. Hyperextension of the low back which compresses the degenerated zygoapophyseal joints is usually uncomfortable and causes low back pain.

The diagnosis of degenerative changes associated with chronic discogenic disease is made from the history of recurrent episodic periods of pain and limitation interspaced with periods of being totally asymptomatic. The examination during the asymptomatic period is often unrewarding except to discover segments of the vertebral column that have not regained their full physiologic movement or to reveal other aspects, such as limited hip joint range of motion, poor muscle tone, limited flexibility, improper use of the back, a short leg of significant difference, or a person whose entire psychological attitude predisposes to further acute attacks.

NERVE ROOT ENTRAPMENT DUE TO INTERVERTEBRAL FORAMINAL CLOSURE

Many patients in later decades of life experience radicular pain of a sciatic nature that cannot be attributed to a disc herniation. These are

178

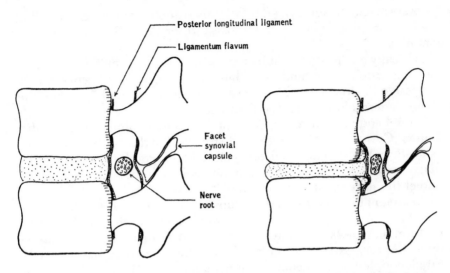

Posterior longitudinal ligament

Ligamentum flavum

Facet synovial capsule

Nerve root

FIGURE 118. Intervertebral foraminal impingement in disc degeneration and spondylosis. The drawing at left shows the normal relationship of two vertebrae adequately spearated by a normal disc. The foramen is open and the merging nerve root free. The drawing at right depicts the foraminal narrowing due to osteophyte impingement and posterior articular closure with synovial irritation. Movement is obviously restricted, and further nerve root pinch can be pictured by extension of this functional unit.

patients who frequently have nondiagnostic myelograms and have negative surgical explorations for a herniated disc.

Patients with this possibility have severe subjective radicular pain and on examination have a positive SLR test. The neurologic examination can demonstrate a single root involvement of both motor and sensory nature, but often, other than a positive Laségue (SLR) test, only minimal objective neurologic signs.[7]

These patients have closure or narrowing of the intervertebral foramina due to:

1. Approximation of the pedicles resulting from narrowing of the intervertebral disc.
2. Osteophyte formation in the ventral aspect of the foramen, called "spurs" (see Fig. 118).
3. Hypertrophic degenerative arthritic changes of the zygoapophyseal joints (facets).
4. Thickening of the ligamentum flavum.

Pain with numbness or paresthesiae in the distribution of the nerve root (dermatome) or weakness in that root distribution (myotome) can

179

be present and be aggravated by slightly extending or hyperextending the lumbar spine. Increase in lordosis further closes the intervertebral foramina.

Typically any posture that increases the lordosis is found to produce pain (e.g., prolonged standing, fatigue, walking, or reaching overhead). Excessive flexion is capable of stretching the nerve and dura over the tissues encroaching upon the foramen.

Lateral and oblique x-ray views of the lumbar spine may be confirmatory. Currently CAT scans can clearly outline the extent of foramina as well as the spinal canal adequacy. Myelography may fail to be diagnostic as the dye column may not extend sufficiently laterally to depict the nerve root entrapment.[8,9,10]

Treatment that decreases the lordosis, such as exercise with or without a brace or corset, improving the posture, and avoiding incriminating posture, may be helpful (see Chapter 5). When pain is intractable or there is progressive neurologic deficit, foraminotomy may be indicated, coupled with decompression surgery.

SPINAL STENOSIS

Many patients in later years develop symptoms of leg pain similar to vascular occlusive disease of the lower extremities as a result of narrowing of the spinal canal. As these claudication symptoms *are not* caused by peripheral vascular disease, they have been termed *pseudo-claudication.*

Recent studies have clearly shown that these symptoms and findings are attributable to narrowing of the lumbar spine canal, a condition termed *spinal stenosis.*[11] (Figs. 119 and 120).

Spinal stenosis causing "neurogenic intermittent claudication"[12] or intermittent ischemia of the cauda equina[13] may result from a herniated lumbar disc, hypertrophic ridging into the spinal canal, spondylolisthesis, post-fusion bony extrusion, Paget's disease, or extradural tumor.

The number of vertebral segments involved may vary from one level to the entire lumbar spine but appear mostly at L_{3-4} and then at the L_{4-5} level.

Many patients develop symptoms from the prolonged lordotic posture as well as from prolonged walking and are relieved by lumbar flexion such as bending forward or assuming a "squat" position.

Extension of the lumbar spine (increased lordosis) causes protrusion of the intervertebral discs dorsally with displacement of the equinal roots.[14] In the extended (lordotic) posture, the length of the canal is decreased and the caudal roots shorten and "bunch," thus also being compressed in the narrowed canal. In an excessive lordotic position, myelogram dye is blocked and resumes flow with lumbar flexion.[15]

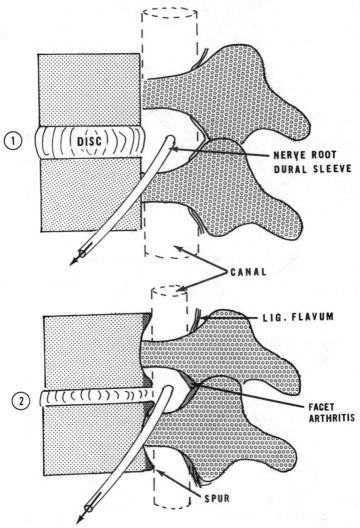

FIGURE 119.   Spondylosis and spinal stenosis. 1. Normal functional unit. 2. Narrowing of intervertebral disc, approximation of adjacent pedicles, spur formation, facet arthritis with resultant narrowing of spinal canal (*broken lines*) and the intervertebral foramen.

The basis of claudication from spinal stenosis consists of the following factors:

1. Neural impulses through the cauda equina to the contracting muscles of that root dilate their radicular arteries.[16]
2. Actively conducting nerve roots require oxygen in competition with the muscles.
3. There is relative ischemia in addition to mechanical nerve obstruction.

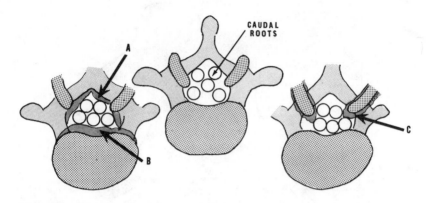

FIGURE 120. Spinal stenosis. The central drawing depicts a normal canal with adequate space for the cauda equina. The drawing at left reveals encroachment from changes in the neural arch (A) and vertebral body osteophytes. The drawing at right reveals degenerative arthritic changes of facets. Usually all factors have involvement in canal stenosis.

The symptoms of this syndrome usually follow a cycle of exercise-pain-rest-relief. There are basic differences in pseudoclaudication that distinguish this condition from aortoiliac occlusive vascular disease:

	Aortoiliac Occlusive Vascular Disease	*Pseudoclaudication/Spinal Stenosis*
Pain site:	Hips, thighs, and buttocks-progress to calf (or in reverse direction)	Lumbar spine and buttocks Pain may occur from prolonged standing or lying with back "arched."
Onset:	After walking a long distance	After walking up inclines
Pain description:	Aching, squeezing, cramping quality increases with walking. Rarely paresthesis or "weakness"	Onset may be tingling, weakness, or clumsiness. "Pain" may be minimal, often numbness or burning, not "cramping."
Relief:	Fast relief by ceasing to walk. Slowing walk decreases onset or severity.	Must sit down and assume flexed trunk posture.
Impotence:	Frequent	May take 20 to 30 minutes for relief
Peripheral pulses:	May disappear after walking Loud bruits, frequently pale legs after walking, no neurologic findings	Saddle distribution of numbness frequent SLR may not be present, and cough may not increase radicular pain. After prolonged walking, pain may occur from SLR. Ankle jerk may be absent after exercise.

The mechanism by which neurogenic claudication is caused is not known. In all probability the symptoms are caused by anoxia of the nerve trunks. This anoxia is probably due to buildup of cerebrospinal fluid pressure behind the obstruction. As cerebrospinal fluid has been shown to flow along the spinal nerve from the point of vertebral exit, compression at the caudal equina upon the venules there could cause ischemia.[17,18]

The diagnosis is suggested by the history and proper examination. Confirmatory x-ray findings are seen on special oblique views, CAT scan, and myelogram.

Treatment

Nonoperative treatment should always be attempted first for relief and for confirmation of diagnosis. Treatment is very similar to the usual mechanical low back etiology syndrome: rest, analgesics, and local modalities. Conservative treatment stresses chiefly the need to decrease the lumbar lordosis with postural exercises, external support, and job counseling as well as posture activity modification.

Surgical intervention is to be considered when:

1. Daily activities are unacceptably restricted or pain is intolerable in spite of adequate conservative treatment. (Daily activities being curtailed reflect a walking distance of 50 yards, sitting time of 30 minutes, night leg cramps interfering with sleep, etc.)
2. Progressive neurologic deficit, such as motor weakness of quadriceps, causes the knee to "buckle" or results in ankle dorsiflexion paresis.
3. Bladder dysfunction is attributable to a neurogenic cause.[19]

The predictable prognosis of surgical decompression must be carefully discussed with the patient. Complete relief of pain is not assured, nor is marked improvement in functional activities predictable. Prevention of further disability, lessening of pain, and improvement in daily function are the major objectives. It is mandatory, therefore, that a carefully documented evaluation of incapacitation (activities of daily living) be made before treatment and repeated after treatment, whether conservative or surgical.

ARACHNOIDITIS

In 1974, 2614 neurosurgeons in the United States performed 117,630 surgical procedures for lumbar disc herniation. There are no comparable statistics on how many were performed by orthopedic surgeons. It is estimated that 10 to 40 percent were long-term failures.

Many long-term failures are attributed to lumbosacral arachnoiditis. This is difficult to determine and verify as the diagnosis of arachnoiditis requires direct observation by surgical exploration or by unequivocal myelographic changes.

Arachnoiditis is essentially inflammation of the arachnoid. The arachnoid is a nonvascular membrane composed of fibrous and elastic tissue that envelopes the cord and is noncellular.

The presenting signs and symptoms of this entity are sparce. They are usually complaints of constant low back pain with or without leg pain markedly aggravated by activity. Definite motor weakness is rare. Patients demonstrate a positive straight-leg raising and complain that their gait requires a short step to avoid pain. Examination reveals tenderness of the sciatic nerve at the sciatic notch, limited trunk flexion, and paravertebral muscle spasm.

Numerous etiologies for arachnoiditis have been postulated. These include infection, trauma, foreign bodies, allergic reaction vascular abnormalities, and numerous other causes. More recently chemical reaction to myelographic dye with or without blood has been incriminated. Trauma from the surgical procedure completes the eventual inflammatory reaction of the pia-arachnoid.

Stages have been postulated in the natural evolution of arachnoiditis:

1. Inflammation of the pia-arachnoid with hyperemia and swelling of the nerve roots. At this stage there is little fibroelastic proliferation. Some strands of collagen begin to be deposited between the nerve roots and their pia-arachnoid coating. Around the nerve roots there is a fibrinous exudate with no cellular component.
2. Increase in fibroblastic activity and collagen deposit. The nerve roots no longer swell but they are now adherent to their pia-arachnoid sheath and the sheaths to each other.
3. Adhesive phase marking the end of the inflammatory process. The pia-arachnoid is now markedly thickened as is the collagen deposit. The nerve roots having been ischemic now atrophy. If the subarachnoid space becomes involved as well as the roots, a fourth phase evolves[20] (Fig. 121).

Diagnosis is suggested by intractable pain in the low back and often down the involved leg. There is normal spinal fluid protein and no spinal fluid cytology. Confirmation of the diagnosis is accomplished by myelography and/or exploration.

Treatment remains largely unsatisfactory or its benefit limited. Lysis under microscopic surgical procedure has been advocated but with limited success and often with postoperative scar formation.[21] In-

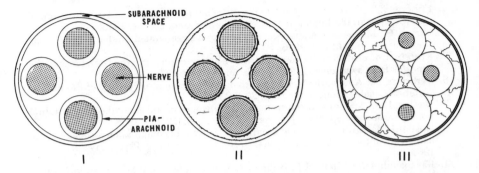

FIGURE 121. Arachnoiditis: natural evolution. I. The nerve roots with their enveloping pia-arachnoid in the normal state. II. The roots swell and the pia-arachnoid becomes inflamed and thickened. There are small adhesions between the roots and the arachnoid. III. The roots are atrophic and the pia-arachnoid is adherent with fibrous and collagen strands. The subarachnoid space is thickened as well.

tradural steroids have been used,[22] as has deep x-ray therapy. The correction of contributory pathology such as spinal stenosis or disc herniation frequently restores function in patients and decreases their pain. More recently "spinal forceful flexion" under anesthesia has been of value. A spinal anesthetic to the T_8 sensory level is administered. Once the anesthetic is achieved, the patient's knees are brought to the chest individually, gently but firmly. If there are no arachnoidal adhesions, this maneuver will not be restricted. If there are adhesions, the movement will be restricted and when stretched a "give" will be experienced.

When an adhesion is torn, the patient experiences a sensation in the cervical region but no pain. Immediately after the stretch, the roots move more freely in their foramina and SLR is increased. Following the procedure under anesthesia, the patient must do flexion exercises routinely.

In cases of intractable pain, posterior column stimulation, transcutaneous nerve stimulation, and other procedures used for chronic pain should be considered.[23,24,25]

REFERENCES

1. Püschel, J.: Wassergehalt normalen und degeneraten zwischen Wirbelscheiben. Beitr. Pathol. 84:123-130, 1930.
2. Friberg, S., and Hirsch, C.: Anatomical and clinical studies in lumbar disc degeneration. Acta Orthop. Scand. 19:222-242, 1949.
3. Hirsch, C.: Studies on the pathology of low back pain. J. Bone Joint Surg. 41-B(2):237-243, 1959.

4. Farfan, H.F.: Mechanical Disorders of the Low Back. Lea & Febiger, Philadelphia, 1973, pp. 63-92.
5. Friberg, S., and Hirsch, C.: On late results of operative treatment for intervertebral disc prolapse in the lumbar region. Acta Chir. Scand. 93:161, 1946.
6. Hirsch, C.: Mechanical responses in normal and degenerated lumbar discs. J. Bone Joint Surg. 38-A:242-243, 1956.
7. Epstein, J.A., et al.: Sciatica caused by nerve root entrapment in the lateral recess: the superior facet syndrome. J. Neurosurg. 36:584-589, 1972.
8. Verbriest, H.: A radicular syndrome from developmental narrowing of the lumbar vertebral canal. J. Bone Joint Surg. 26-B:230-237, 1954.
9. Hadley, L.A.: Apophyseal subluxation: disturbances in and about the intervertebral foramen causing back pain. J. Bone Joint Surg. 18:428-433, 1936.
10. Epstein, J.A., Epstein, B.S., and Lavine, L.: Nerve root compression associated with narrowing of the lumbar spinal canal. J. Neurol. Neurosurg. Psychiatry 25:165-176, 1962.
11. Kavanaugh, G.J., Svien, H.J., Holman, C.B., and Johnson, R.M.: "Pseudoclaudication" syndrome produced by compression of the cauda equina. J.A.M.A. 206(11):2477-2481, 1968.
12. Evans, J.G.: Neurogenic intermittent claudication. Br. Med. J. 2:985-987, 1964.
13. Blau, J.N., and Logue, V.: Intermittent claudication of the cauda equina: an unusual syndrome resulting from central protrusion of a lumbar intervertebral disc. Lancet 1:1081-1086, 1961.
14. Breig, A.: Biomechanics of the Central Nervous System: Some Basic Normal and Pathological Phenomena. Year Book Medical Publishers, Chicago, 1960.
15. Ehni, G.: Spondylatic cauda equina radiculopathy. Texas State J. Med. 61:746-752, 1965.
16. Blau, J.N., and Rushworth, G.: Observations on the blood vessels of the spinal cord with their responses to motor activity. Brain 81:354-363, 1958.
17. Wilson, C.B.: Significance of the small lumbar spine canal—cauda equina compression syndrome due to spondylosis. J. Neurosurg. 31(5):499-506, 1969.
18. Steer, J.C., and Horney, F.D.: Evidence for passage of cerebrospinal fluid along spinal nerves. Can. Med. Assoc. J. 98:71-74, 1968.
19. Lee, C.K., Hanson, H.T., and Weiss, A.B.: Developmental lumbar spine stenosis— pathology and surgical treatment. Spine 3(3):246-255, 1978.
20. Burton, C.V.: Lumbosacral arachnoiditis. Spine 3(1):24-30, 1978.
21. Johnston, J.D.H., and Matheny, J.B.: Microscopic lysis of lumbar adhesive arachnoiditis. Spine 3(1):36, 1978.
22. Feldman, S.: Effect of intrathecal hydrocortisone on adhesive arachnoiditis and cerebrospinal fluid pleocytosis: an experimental study. Neurology 25:256, 1960.
23. Howland, W.J., and Curry, J.L.: Pantopaque arachnoiditis: experimental study of blood as an attenuating agent and corticosteroids as an ameliorating agent. Acta Radiol. Diagn. 5:1032-1041, 1966.
24. Brodsky, A.E.: Cauda equina arachnoiditis. Spine 3(1):51-60, 1978.
25. Wood, K.M.: New approaches to treatment of back pain. Western J. Med. 130(4):394-398, 1979.

CHAPTER 8

Miscellaneous Low Back Conditions and Their Relationship to Low Back Discomfort and Disability

Numerous conditions of the lumbosacral spine are frequently mentioned as causes of low back discomfort and disability. A complete dissertation on these conditions is not within the scope of this text, but no treatise on low back pain would be complete without at least a mention of those most common. These conditions must be considered in the differential diagnosis when they are found to be present, and the symptoms of the patient must be attributed in some part to their presence.

SPONDYLOLISTHESIS

Spondylolisthesis is a condition of forward subluxation of the body of one vertebra on the vertebra below it. The term is derived from the Greek word *olistheses* which means a slipping or falling. The condition of spondylolisthesis is not limited to any specific segment of the vertebral column but most commonly occurs as a displacement of the last lumbar vertebra (L_5) over the body of the sacrum. Whenever a vertebra slips forward on the one below, from any cause, the term spondylolisthesis may be applied.

In the lumbar spine the superior vertebra reposes upon its immediate inferior vertebra upon an inclined plane. This is particularly noted at the L_{4-5} and the L_5-S_1 level. Due to the lordosis, angulation decreases at L_{3-4} and may be reversed more cephalad.

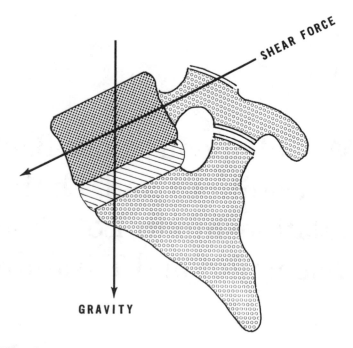

FIGURE 122. Gravitational forces acting upon the lumbosacral joint. The fifth lumbar residing upon the inclined sacral plane tends to glide due to shear force and gravity. Forward gliding is prevented by the facets, ligaments, and annular fibers.

There is a tendency for the superior to glide upon the inferior by gravitational forces (Fig. 122). Normally sliding is prevented by the mechanical relationship of the articular facets and their ligaments. Further support is added by the alignment and the adequacy of the longitudinal ligaments, the integrity of the disc annular fibers, and the intradiscal pressure that maintains the tautness within the functional unit.

Defects or impairment of any of the supporting structures can lead to listhesis. Spondylolisthesis has been classified according to etiology into five types.

Type I (Isthmic). In isthmic spondylolisthesis there is a defect in the pars interarticularis. This defect may be a separation of the pars due to fracture or merely an elongation of the pars without separation (Fig. 123).

Type II (Congenital). In congenital spondylolisthesis the posterior elements are anatomically inadequate due to developmental deficiency. This occurs rarely.

Type III (Degenerative). In degenerative spondylolisthesis the facets and/or the supporting ligaments undergo degenerative changes,

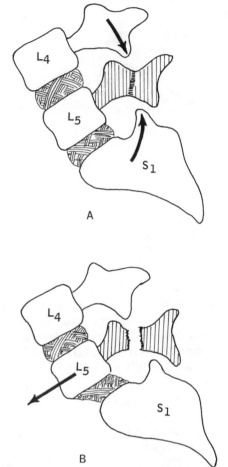

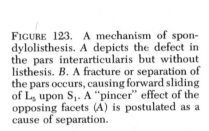

FIGURE 123. A mechanism of spondylolisthesis. *A* depicts the defect in the pars interarticularis but without listhesis. *B*. A fracture or separation of the pars occurs, causing forward sliding of L_5 upon S_1. A "pincer" effect of the opposing facets (*A*) is postulated as a cause of separation.

A

B

allowing listhesis. There is no pars defect, and the condition increases with aging (Fig. 124).

Type IV (Elongated Pedicles). In Type IV spondylolisthesis the length of the neural arch elongates to allow listhesis. This is essentially an isthmic type. Traction forces are apparently contributory.

Type V (Destructive Disease). Type V spondylolisthesis is due to metastatic disease, tuberculosis, or other bone diseases that may change the structure of the supporting tissues.

The presence of a defect or a minor degree of listhesis on an x-ray does not necessarily imply that the patient is symptomatic. Listhesis, however, is becoming recognized with increasing frequency and is being considered more significant as a cause of chronic disabling backache. A congenital defect can exist through an entire lifetime without

189

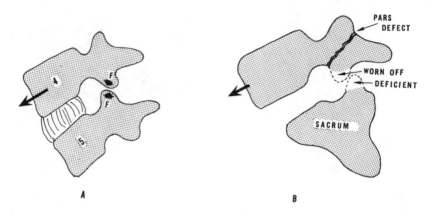

FIGURE 124. Type III spondylolisthesis. *A* depicts the facet factor that prevents listhesis (F-F). *B*. Facets are worn and permit listhesis. The pars defect is intact and does not cause listhesis.

the patient's awareness of its presence. Trauma, however, is probably the inciting cause of symptomatology. Statistically, 70 percent of spondylolisthesis occurs at the fifth vertebra, 25 percent at the fourth, and only 4 percent at higher levels.

Studies have claimed that progression of listhesis is unusual after age 20, with stability predictable between ages 20 and 70. Recent studies[1-4] refute this with the conclusion that listhesis above the lumbosacral level (L_{4-5})

1. has a higher incidence of neurologic signs;
2. has a higher incidence of spinal stenosis due in part to excessive cartilaginous mass at the pseudoarthrosis;
3. has a higher incidence of further slipping in later life, which is rare at L_5-S_1.

Symptoms

The chief complaint in spondylolisthesis is that of backache accompanied by referred pain to the sacroiliac joints. Pain may radiate into the hips, thighs, and even into the feet (10 percent), but usually symptoms are in the low back area with numbness or "tingling" noted in the legs.

Stiffness of the back is claimed, and limited forward flexion of the lumbar spine is noted during the examination. Muscle "spasm" is frequent, and patients claim discomfort from lifting or bending.

The clinical diagnosis is suggested by inspection and palpation of the back in which a depression above the sacrum is noted as well as an

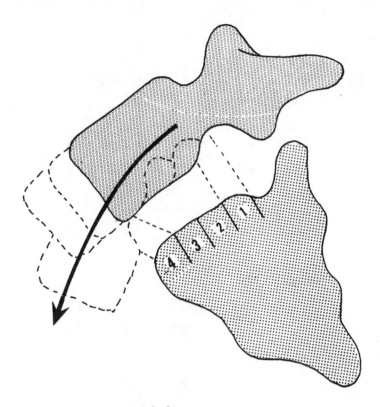

FIGURE 125. Grading of spondylolisthesis.

accentuated lumbar lordosis. Rectal and proctoscopic examination may disclose a hard, fixed mass in front of the sacrum. Percussion (by the examiner) over the lumbosacral joint may elicit pain.

In young people, ages 11 to 17, spondylolisthesis can be associated with tight hamstring muscles. These patients present a peculiar gait due to posterior tilting of the pelvis,[2] lumbar lordosis, spinal stiffness, and flexed hips and knees. All have limited straight-leg raising to approximately 45 degrees bilaterally. Most are negative neurologically and have no urinary tract dysfunction.

The cause of the hamstring tightness remains unknown but has been attributed to cauda equinal traction with irritation to the nerves to the hamstring muscles.

The condition of the neural arch may involve a defect in the pars articularis, a fracture, elongation of the arch, or severe angulation, all of which can be noted on plain x-ray films. The width of the spinal canal can be estimated and actually measured.

Lateral views of the lower lumbar vertebrae and the sacrum reveal the degree of subluxation which can be graded (Fig. 125).

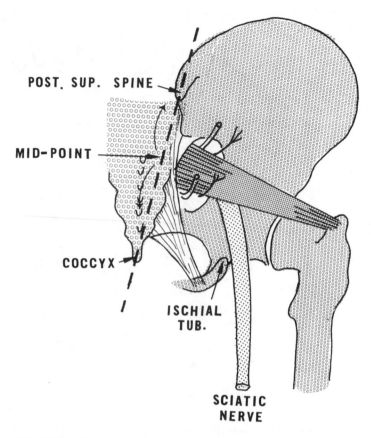

POST. SUP. SPINE

MID-POINT

COCCYX

ISCHIAL
TUB.

SCIATIC
NERVE

FIGURE 126. Piriformis muscle. Anatomical relationship of the sciatic nerve to the piriformis muscle is noted.

Treatment

Nonsurgical treatment of spondylolisthesis consists of instructing the patient in methods of decreasing the lumbar lordosis. Recumbency with flexion of the lumbar spine is indicated in acute cases. Traction is of value, especially suspension by the legs from an overhead frame.

Plaster casting can be useful to immobilize the lumbar spine in a pelvic tilted position for a period of 6 weeks. This measure may then be followed by use of a brace to insure the same posture. Exercises done within and after bracing and casting are valuable.

The vast majority of cases of spondylolisthesis can be treated conservatively. Only when the patient fails to respond is surgery indicated, more often in the young child or young adult than in the older adult.

Surgery involves posterior fusion from L_4-S_1, L_5 to the sacrum, or anterior interbody fusion with or without laminectomy. The proper procedure depends upon the judgment and experience of the surgeon.

In cases of childhood spondylolisthesis there is marked disagreement as to the best manner of treatment, and most surgical procedures (e.g., laminectomy with or without fusion to reduce the spondylolesthesis) have resulted in only limited benefit.

PIRIFORM SYNDROME

Pain of a sciatic type has been attributed to a myofasciitis of the piriform muscle.[5] Pain is complained of in the region of the hip, tail bone, buttocks, and down the leg in a sciatic distribution. Because a high percentage of patients are women there is often associated dyspareunia.

The piriform muscle, an external rotater of the hips, arises from inside the pelvis in the region of the sacrum and the sacroiliac joint. It passes laterally out of the sciatic notch to insert upon the greater trochanter of the femur. The sciatic nerve passes between two bellies of the muscle (Fig. 126).

Description of the pain is usually imprecise, and the diagnosis is suspected because there is no evidence of the "sciatica" originating from the lumbosacral spine, nor are there objective neurologic findings other than an equivocally positive straight-leg raising.

There are no causative factors consistently elicited in the piriform syndrome. Occasionally the patient recalls an incident of stress or trauma to the hip joint, such as twisting while walking, having the legs excessively abducted while lifting, or standing too long in an awkward position. Usually no significant history can be elicited.

On physical examination the lumbar spine has normal range of motion. Straight-leg raising may be restricted and painful, but only when the leg is simultaneously internally rotated. Pain and weakness is noted on resisted abduction and external rotation of the thigh.[6] This latter test can be elicited with the patient seated, hips and knees flexed at right angles, and asked to separate the legs while they are resisted.

Rectal or pelvic examination usually reveals tenderness over the lateral pelvic wall proximal to the ischial spine.

X-rays of the hip joint and the lumbosacral spine are nonspecific. Laboratory tests are not diagnostic.

Treatment requires direct local injection into the piriform muscle of an anesthetic agent. There are two avenues of administration: by the vaginal route directly into the tender region of the muscle or by inserting a 3-inch spinal needle through the buttocks and the sacral notch toward the tender spot located by the gloved finger that, rectally, is on the painful tender area.

The patient is awake during the injection and notifies the physician if the sciatic nerve is touched. Being conscious, the patient can inform the physician of the exact site of tenderness and relief from the anesthetic agent.

SACRALIZED TRANSVERSE PROCESS

Sacralization of a transverse process, a congenitally long transverse process forming a pseudoarthrosis at its point of contact with the sacrum or the ilium, is capable of causing low back pain and sciatica. The usual level of the elongated transverse process is the fifth lumbar vertebra, and the pseudoarthrosis is found at its tip and at the point in contact with the ipsilateral ilium.

Pain resulting from movement at the pseudoarthrosis will be caused by or be aggravated mostly during the movement of lateral flexion of the trunk, as contrasted with discogenic disease in which pain occurs during anterior-posterior movement.

Sciatic pain, when it occurs because of this condition, localizes at a level of the L_4 root or a higher root in the area in which the nerve root is irritated (Fig. 127). Pain is more sharply localized at the site of sacralization. Motor, sensory, and reflex changes are rare, even in the presence of subjective sciatica.

The large transverse process and its sacral pseudoarthrosis must be visualized on x-ray film even to consider the feasibility of this diagnosis. The possible occurrence of a herniated lumbar disc with radiculitis in a patient whose x-rays reveal a large transverse process and a suggested pseudoarthrosis must be kept in mind.

SACROILIAC JOINT PATHOLOGY

The sacroiliac joint is the *bête noire* of low back pain syndromes, avidly claimed as prevalent by some and violently disclaimed by others.[7]

Goldthwaite and Osgood introduced the concept of "sacroiliac sprain" as a common cause of low back pain in 1905. This is still advocated, but many feel that pain over the sacroiliac area is referred there from elsewhere. Bourdillon[8] notes:

> The range of motion in the sacroiliac joint is small and its demonstration by direct palpitation is both difficult and unconvincing . . . Indeed the existence and importance of sacroiliac mobility is still a subject of argument.

A method of testing and simultaneously treating lesions of the sacroiliac joint is by using the strong and flexible capsular ligaments of the

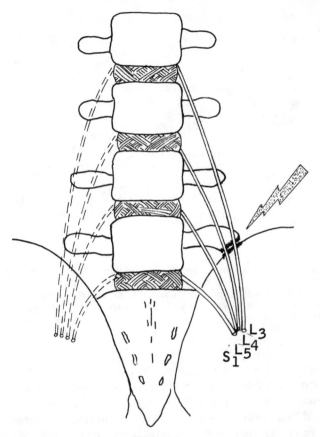

FIGURE 127. Sacralization of the transverse process. The elongated left transverse process of the fifth lumbar vertebra forms a pseudoarthrosis at its point of contact with the sacral wing. The passage over the area of pseudoarthrosis of the L_{3-4} nerve roots irritates the contiguous branches. The mechanism of pain due to mechanical irritation on left lateral flexion can be visualized.

hip joints upon the pelvis. With the hips externally rotated and adducted, extension posteriorly rotates the pelvis forward and downward. The pelvis can be rotated backward by placing the hip in slight abduction and internally rotated then extended. These movements allegedly test mobility of the sacroiliac joints. A forceful thrust in those directions upon reaching the full range of motion is claimed to be therapeutic.[9]

The sacroiliac joint is an extremely stable joint marked by reinforcement of powerful ligaments anteriorly and posteriorly (Fig. 128). Also the articular surfaces are so curved and sigmoid in their direction that

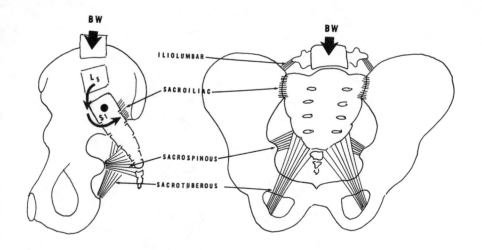

FIGURE 128. Forces acting on the pelvis. The body weight is imposed upon the fifth lumbar vertebra which lies on the sacrum. This weight is transmitted through the sacrum, across the sacroiliac joints, through the ilia, into the acetabula, and finally to the femora. The two compressive forces of the femoral heads are resisted by the superimposed pubic strut. When the body weight is borne in the sitting position, the forces tend to spread the ilia. This is resisted by the symphysis pubis and the sacroiliac ligaments.

movement must be limited (Fig. 129). After age 45 it has been shown that 35 percent of the population has ossified immobile sacroiliac joints.

During pregnancy there is "softening" with elasticity of the sacroiliac joint ligaments. Other than that violent trauma to the "pelvic rim" is necessary to cause sacroiliac joint damage (Fig. 130). The damage to the sacroiliac joint is in conjunction with fracture of the pelvic "ring" or a simultaneous dislocation of the symphysis pubis (Fig. 131).

Trauma to these "ring" structures causes

1. Tenderness over the sacroiliac joint. Usually the lower third of the joint is palpated below the posterior inferior iliac spine.
2. Tenderness of the symphysis pubis.
3. Stress upon the sacroiliac joints and bilateral compression of the iliac crest. With the patient lying on his side, manual direct pressure downward upon the superior iliac crest will cause pain over the sacroiliac joint.
4. Pain on hyperextension of the hip joint on the affected side. This determination, the Gaenslen test, is no longer considered specific for the sacroiliac joint and stresses the hip joint. Also it hyperextends the lumbar spine and can cause referred pain from L_{4-5} or L_5-S_1 intervertebral joints.

196

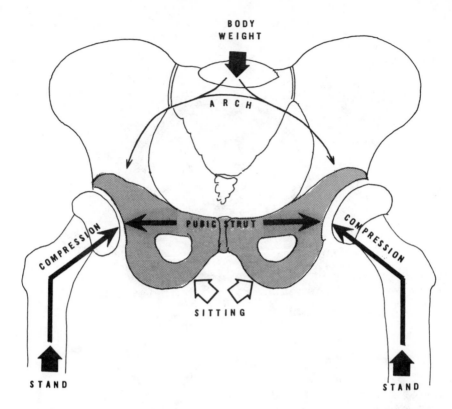

FIGURE 129.   Ligamentous support of the pelvis. The side view of the pelvis indicates the stress of the superincumbent body upon the fifth lumbar vertebra. The downward pressure initiates a rotation about the axis at S_1 with depression of the upper sacral structure and posterior movement of the lower sacrum. This rotation is resisted by the sacrospinous and sacrotuberous ligaments. The front view shows these ligaments and the sacroiliac ligaments that firmly support the posterior border of the pelvic rim.

    5. Resisted abduction of the hip joint with patient lying on his side (Fig. 132).

    Lesser trauma upon the pelvis of the female during the last months of pregnancy can cause minor subluxation of the sacroiliac joints. During these months the expected parturition causes a hormonal ligamentous laxity that permits enlargement of the pelvic ring. Symptoms are those of pain and tenderness over the sacroiliac joints with radiation toward the greater trochanters and down the anterior aspect of the thighs. The findings are as stated above.

    Treatment during pregnancy may afford relief by a trochanteric belt fitted about the pelvis below the iliac crest. Steroid anesthetic injections into the sacroiliac joint are of value.

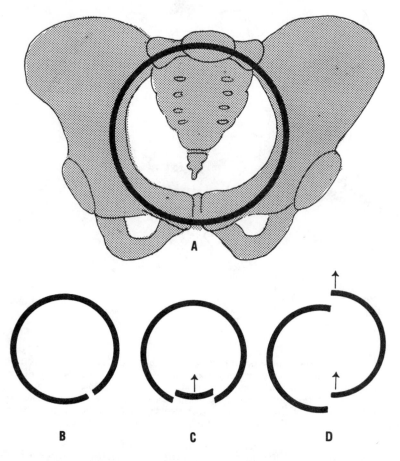

FIGURE 130. Pelvic ring. The pelvic ring is bounded laterally by the ilia, anteriorly by the pubic rami, and posteriorly by the sacrum and the sacroiliac joints. An intact ring of great strength is thus formed. The lower drawings depict the various types of fracture-dislocations that may occur and their effects upon the integrity of the ring.

Trauma that at the onset gives no indication of separation of sacroiliac joints and/or the symphysis pubis may subsequently reveal x-ray evidence of that injury.

Sacroiliac instability may be demonstrated by anterior posterior x-ray views of the pelvis of the patient standing upon a small step, standing on one leg and the dependent leg weighted and dangling. Separation of the involved joint may be elicited.

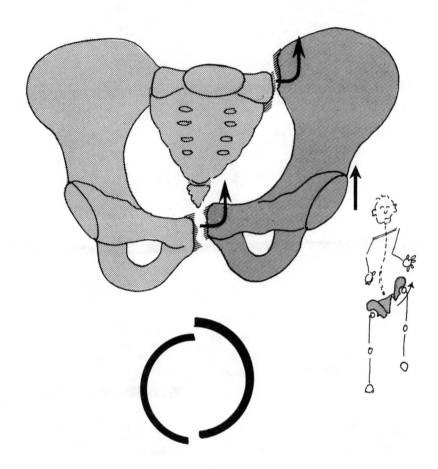

FIGURE 131. Combined sacroiliac and symphysis pubis separation. Injury resulting in combined separation of the symphysis pubis and the sacroiliac joints disrupts the pelvic ring. The fractured segment rotates posteriorly behind the sacrum and elevates. The involved leg is "shortened."

Sacroiliac inflammation is noted early or subsequently in rheumatoid spondylitis (Marie-Strumpell spondylitis). HLA-W27 is positive, whereas a latex fixation may be negative. Other tests of rheumatoid disease are noted.

Patients are usually male in their second or third decade. There is often a genetic factor where HLA-W27 may be found in members of the family who may not have the disease.

199

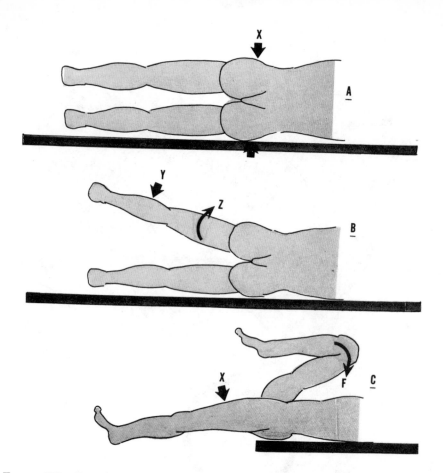

FIGURE 132. Sacroiliac tests. *A.* Direct pressure upon the iliac crest with patient side-lying on a firm surface. *B.* Resisted abduction of the involved side with hip extension. *C.* Hyperextension of the hip on the side of the painful sacroiliac joint.

Patients with spondylitis may initially have negative x-rays but they have low back pain with limited flexibility and early have restricted respiratory inspiration (decreased chest expansion). There may also be tenderness over the sternomanubrial joints.

In a young male with these symptoms, periodic x-rays will gradually reveal a "fuzziness" of the sacroiliac joints. Initially, oblique views of the sacroiliac joints may show a widening of the joints (due to subendochondral bone softening); then gradual sclerosis to alternate ossification. As the disease progresses, diagnostic changes appear in the entire vertebral column as well as changes in the cardiovascular system.

Certain significant findings and symptoms can indicate the possibility of rheumatoid spondylitis. Ultimately the diagnosis is as follows:

1. Usually male;
2. Age of onset, 20 to 30 years;
3. Aching "stiff" back;
4. Limited lumbar flexibility;
5. Decreased chest expansion;
6. Normal blood studies with even sedimentation rate normal but HLA-W27 antigen present;
7. "Positive" sacroiliac signs;
8. "Fuzziness" on x-rays of sacroiliac joints;
9. Concavity of the manubrial-sternal joint.

Treatment is essentially symptomatic with utilization of anti-inflammatory drugs, but primarily to minimize or prevent deformity. These deformities are excessive dorsal kyphosis with compensatory cervical lordosis and hip flexion contracture. Nonsurgical treatment[10,11] involves the following measures:

1. Proper sleeping posture on a firm, flat bed without pillow. Frequent sleeping or lying in prone position.
2. Posture exercises with upper back hyperextension (performed with avoidance of lumbar hyperextension).
3. Breathing exercises to increase or maintain rib cage excursion, as well as instruction in abdominothoracic breathing.
4. Range of motion exercises for hips and knees to prevent flexion limitation and contractures.
5. Periodic rest periods with avoidance of fatigue.
6. Bracing or corseting if combined with exercises. A night-time posterior mold plastic cast to insure thoracic extension and lumbar flexion has value if made tolerable.

Surgery is a corrective procedure when the deformities are cosmetically unacceptable or are causing functional loss or when they threaten respiratory or neurologic damage. These procedures are essentially osteotomies at the cervical thoracic junction or the thoracolumbar junction. Hip flexion contractures may also need to be released.

SPINAL INFECTIONS

Infection of the spine, although rare, must always be considered in the differential diagnosis of low back pain. Infection may affect the vertebral body, causing an osteomyelitis, or may affect the intervertebral disc.

Vertebral osteomyelitis has many causative factors. It may result as a hematogenous spread through arterial or venous routes, secondary often to pelvic inflammatory disease or genitourinary tract infection.

Vertebral osteomyelitis is mostly caused by a staphylococcus. The onset is insidious and usually proceeds into a chronic course. Diabetics appear to be especially susceptible.

Usually two adjacent vertebrae and their intervening disc are involved. The body or bodies may undergo destruction and collapse. Abscess formation may result with possible neurologic involvement.

The infection presents as a "nonspecific backache." Eight to 12 weeks later, x-rays reveal the diagnosis. Pain may be moderate to severe. All movement is painful and there is marked muscular guarding of the paravertebral muscles and the hamstrings. *Percussion over the involved vertebrae is usually exquisitely sensitive, and pain is more severe at night.*

Early laboratory tests are not helpful as the white blood count may not be elevated and the patient not specifically toxic or febrile. Blood cultures often remain negative until the patient develops a severe toxic sequela. The *sedimentation rate is usually markedly elevated,* which should be a warning sign when present.

X-rays become diagnostic in 4 to 6 weeks. There is an early rarefaction of the vertebral end plates with narrowing of the disc space. This can lead to confusion as to whether the initial infection is in the body or the disc. As the disease progresses there is destructive erosion of the vertebral body, always with disc destruction.

Treatment requires isolation of the organism by biopsy or needle aspiration. Antibiotic treatment will depend on sensitivity studies. Bed rest with or without a snug-fitting body cast is indicated, usually for 3 to 6 months. Fusion occurs in 50 percent of patients unless abscess formation results.

Tuberculosis must always be considered as the infectious agent. This is often secondary to tuberculosis elsewhere in the body, such as in the pulmonary or urinary tract. In this infection *the vertebral body undergoes destruction, and the disc remains resistant.*

In tuberculosis there are usually associated constitutional symptoms such as fever, weight loss, sweats, and malaise. Here too the sedimentation rate is elevated with no significant elevated white blood count. Cultures may be diagnostic but may take weeks to grow.

Treatment of tuberculous vertebral ostomyelitis requires immobilization, but surgical debridement is usually indicated.

INTERVERTEBRAL DISC-SPACE INFECTION

Infectious "discitis" is increasingly more common. The variety that is secondary to surgery to the spine following discectomy should be suspected when some 2 to 8 weeks after surgery the patient develops severe low back pain, marked rigidity, and local tenderness. Pain is usually "excruciating," restricting any movement and present at night as well as during the day. Sedimentation is usually markedly elevated.

X-rays reveal gradual narrowing of the disc space with haziness and sclerosing of the vertebral end plates. The end plates gradually become irregular and lose their contour. The vertebral bodies also gradually undergo destruction. A scan reveals a "hot spot."

Biopsy or needle aspiration, performed under x-ray guidance to assure that the biopsy needle is in the disc, will often culture the organism and permit more specific antibiotic therapy.

Discitis of an infectious type occurs following bacteremia secondary to urinary tract infection, with or without instrumentation such as catheterization or cystoscopy. Inasmuch as numerous drugs are self-administered intravenously with improper sterile technique, the "addict" is a frequent sufferer of infectious discitis. Treatment requires antibiotic treatment and the same immobilization as is indicated for vertebral osteomylitis.

BONE TUMORS

Bone tumors of the vertebral bodies must always be suspect in chronic, persistent, resistant low back pains that are unrelated to activities or even more often are present at rest and at night.

Primary bone tumors are rare, but secondary or metastatic invasions are more frequent. These are beyond the scope of this presentation.

Metabolic bone disease often presents as low back pain and is suspect by age and by vague symptoms and findings. The condition is generally confirmed by x-ray and laboratory tests.

INTRASPINAL LESION CAUSING SCIATICA

Intraspinal tumors can mimic the history and objective findings of a herniated lumbar disc. This possibility must never be overlooked. The numerous types of intraspinous lesions are frequently listed in medical literature and will not be repeated here. The true nature of a lesion, other than a herniated lumbar disc, cannot be accurately determined from the history or from the neurologic or orthopedic examination alone. Standard routine roentgenograms are not conclusive, nor usually are they even suggestive of such a diagnosis. Only by Pantopaque studies preceded by spinal fluid studies is this type of lesion suggested as a possibility.

The existence of an intraspinal lesion, other than a herniated lumbar

203

disc, should be suspected when (1) there is a failure to respond to conservative treatment and the pain remains intractable or when there is unusual progression of the neurologic signs. This failure to respond even in probable disc trouble should lead to consideration of myelography which may then reveal the tumor. It should also be suspected when (2) a neurogenic type of bladder or bowel dysfunction exists, or when (3) nocturnal pain awakens the patient and when such pain is essentially unrelated to movement, position, or activity, or when (4) the presence of upper motor neuron is involved neurologically. The presence of spasticity, hyperactive reflexes, clonus, and positive Babinski signs all indicate a lesion in the central nervous system and not of the lower neuron type of involvement found in herniated disc disease. Findings not related to a single nerve root level (myotome or dermatome) should also raise doubt regarding a disc as the reason for the symptoms or the findings.

The suspicion of possible cord tumor rather than disc herniation can be confirmed by lumbar puncture, spinal fluid studies, cystometric confirmation tests of bladder function, Pantopaque myelography, and ultimately surgical exploration.

REFERENCES

1. Jackson, A.M., Kirwan, E.O., and Sullivan, M.F.: Lytic spondylolisthesis above the lumbosacral level. Spine 3(3):260-266, 1978.
2. Phalen, G.S., and Dickson, J.A.: Spondylolisthesis and tight hamstrings: Proceedings of the Association of Bone and Joint Surgeons. J. Bone Joint Surg. 38-A:946, 1956.
3. Barash, H.L., Galante, J.O., Lambert, E.N., and Ray, R.D.: Spondylolisthesis and tight hamstrings. J. Bone Joint Surg. 52-A(7):1319-1328, 1970.
4. Meyerding, H.W.: Spondylolisthesis. Surg. Gynecol. Obstet. 54:371-377, 1932.
5. Pace, J.B., and Nagle, D.: Piriform syndrome. Western J. Med. 124:435-439, 1976.
6. Freiburg, A.H.: Sciatica pain and its relief by operation on muscle and fascia. Arch. Surg. 34:337, 1937.
7. Freiburg, A.H., and Vinke, T.A.: Sciatica and the sacroiliac joint. J. Bone Joint Surg. 16:126, 1934.
8. Bourdillon, J.F.: Spinal Manipulation. Appleton-Century-Crofts, New York, 1970.
9. Brooke, R.: The sacroiliac joint. J. Anat. 58:299-305, 1924.
10. Grieve, G.P.: The sacroiliac joint. Physiotherapy 62(12):384-400, 1976.
11. MacNab, I.: Backache. Williams & Wilkins, Baltimore, 1977, pp. 64-79.

BIBLIOGRAPHY

Bailey, W.: Observations on the etiology and frequency of spondylolisthesis and its precursors. Radiology 48:107, 1947.
Craig, W.M., Svien, H.J., Dodge, H.W., and Camp, J.D.: Intraspinal lesions masquerading as protruded lumbar intervertebral disks. J.A.M.A., May 17, 1952, pp. 250-253.
Friberg, S.: Studies on spondylolisthesis. Acta Chir. Scand. 82(Suppl. 55), 1939.
Hanraets, P.R.M.J.: The Degenerative Back. Elsevier, New York, 1959.
Herz, R.: Subfascial fat herniation as a cause of low back pain. Ann. Rheum. Dis. 11(1):30-35, 1952.

Meyerding, H.W.: The low backache and sciatic pain associated with spondylolisthesis and protruded intervertebral disc: incidence and treatment. J. Bone Joint Surg. 23:461, 1941.

Moore, D.C.: Sciatic and femoral nerve block. J.A.M.A., October 11, 1952, pp. 550-554.

Silver, R.A., et al.: Intermittent claudication of neurospinal origin. Arch. Surg. 98:523-529, 1969.

Soren, A.: Spondylolisthesis and allied conditions. 8(1):8-15, 1966.

Teng, P., and Papatheodorou, C.: Lumbar spondylosis with compression of cauda equina. Arch. Neurol. 8:221-229, 1963.

Young, H.H.: Non-neurological lesions simulating protruded intervertebral disk. J.A.M.A. 148(13):1101-1106, 1952.

CHAPTER 9

Chronic Pain

Chronic pain is the most serious disabling disease of humans. Pain can no longer be considered merely a symptom; it may actually be a disease itself.[1] Intractable pain may lead to narcotic addiction, expensive disability, or ill-advised surgery of questionable value.[2] The low back is a focal point of much chronic pain.

Chronic pain is a disease state in which many factors interact with one another—one reinforcing the other—often being initiated by a physical insult,[1] yet being or becoming independent of any continuing physical insult or damage to the body.

Brena[2] has enumerated five sequences seen in chronic pain which he terms the "Five-D Syndrome."

1. Drug: abuse or misuse.
2. Dysfunction: a decrease in function, performance or even the quality of life.
3. Disuse: loss of flexibility, strength, endurance and alternate degeneration.
4. Depression: with significant loss, real or fantasized, reactive depression may result.[3]
5. Disability: inability to perform activities of daily living or pursue gainful employment.

How one thinks of pain depends upon the evaluator's learning, experience, or specialty. The neurologist considers pain a neurophysiologic abnormality which the neurosurgeon approaches surgically or with electrical implantation. The psychiatrist considers chronic pain an emotional response to internal emotional conflict. The behavioral scientist considers chronic pain an emotional response to internal emotional conflict resulting in psychosocial maladjustment with resultant manipulative response. The pharmacologist considers chronic pain a biochemical aberration that can be therapeutically benefited by medication. The orthopedist evaluates chronic pain of the low back on the basis of x-ray and specialized tests which respond to bracing or surgical intervention. The physiatrist attacks the problem diagnostically with electrodiagnostic means and treats with modalities of heat, cold and exercise. All interrelate but chronic pain may develop and refute all theories.

Steinbach[4] classified pain as an abstract concept which the patient describes as a personal sensation of "hurt" that may signal tissue damage aimed to protect the organism from harm.

There are numerous concepts of pain related to neurophysiologic, physiologic, behavioral, or psychiatric bases, but all may well relate to noxious irritation of sensitive tissues within the vertebral column. Chronic pain is essentially prolongation of an acute incidence with additional ramifications.

The neurophysiologic mechanism of pain is undergoing intensive revision. The original concept of specific irritation of definitive nociceptors transmitted through isolated tracts in the cord to isolated pain centers in the brain is no longer accepted.

Bonica[5] classifies *chronic* pain into three groups:

1. persistent peripheral noxious stimulants;
2. neuraxis pain;
3. learned pain behavior.

In his first group he lists long-term medical conditions such as arthritis, herniated disc, and cancer. All these are certainly related to subjective low back pain. In the second group he involves the nervous system: the peripheral nerves, the cord or the brain. Recent neurophysiologic research is clarifying the role of this system in chronic pain. In the third group he classifies the patients who receive reward for being sick or impaired.

There are two major neurophysiologic theories of pain transmission:

1. The *specificity theory* claims that under each sensitive spot there lies a unique nerve terminal which, when stimulated, arouses a specific sensation. This was classified to include touch-sensitive Meissner's corpuscles, cold-sensitive Krause's end bulbs, and heat-sensitive Ruffini's end organs. These end organs have never been histologically or physiologically confirmed nor found to be of a specific modality. More probably, the peripheral nerve endings that transmit sensation are chemoreceptors irritated by variable intensity of stimuli from irritation of tissue within which they reside.

207

2. The *pattern theory* implies a specific sensation, such as pain, as an encoded spatiotemporal transmission. Once a pattern is "set," any stimulation may be similarly interpreted, although difficult to substantiate objectively. There is a relationship between the intensity of the stimulus and the magnitude of sensations. This concept currently is the only application of the specificity theory.

There are two major neurophysiologic transmission systems (Fig. 133):

1. Spinothalamocortical transmission system—involves few neurons, has a short latency, and precisely discriminates intensity and duration.
2. Spinoreticulothalamic transmission system—has complex multisynaptic connections, does not precisely discriminate location, and has a long latency. It projects to the limbic system and is involved in the emotional system.

There are several accepted classifications of nervous fibers:

Fiber A: myelinated afferent, efferent, somatic
Fiber B: myelinated preganglionic and thus sympathetic
Fiber C: unmyelinated somatic, afferent, and/or sympathetic

Fibers A and C transmit pain sensation. A fibers are further divided into (1) alpha (12-21 μ in diameter); (2) beta (8-12 μ); (3) gamma (5-10 μ) which transmit impulses rapidly and localize sensation; (4) delta. As C fibers transmit to the fasciculus proprius on *both sides* and are considered to carry pain sensation, it is possible that pain is transmitted up both sides. The multiplicity and bilaterality of pain-transmitting tracts in the cord probably explain the unpredictability of cordotomy that is performed to control chronic pain.

There is no specificity of nerve fibers and nerve endings that transmit *pain* rather than touch, pressure or temperature. Free nerve endings found everywhere can transmit pain sensation. Spatial and temporal mechanisms must operate in the encoding of pain perception.

In recent years Wahl and Melzack postulated a neurophysiologic concept of a "gate" in the region of the dorsal horn in the spinal cord gray matter (Fig. 134). This concept attempts to clarify the role of specificity versus pattern. The gate theory postulates that the faster-conducting large fibers, which carry mainly touch and proprioception, project to the substantia gelatinosa and then to the T cells. The substantia gelatinosa exerts an inhibitory influence upon the affected fibers. The faster fibers increase the substantia gelatinosa activity, but

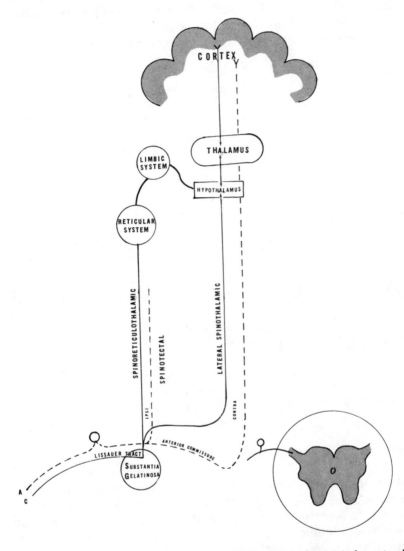

FIGURE 133. Two major neurophysiologic transmission systems: (A) the spinothalamocortic system, which has spatiotemporal localization; and (C) the spinoreticulothalamic system, which has no localization but is involved in emotional (limbic) and avoidance reaction.

the slower C fibers, allegedly related to pain transmission, exert inhibitory influence. Since the slower impulses reach the gate later than the larger fiber impulses, they find the gate closed. How the receptor endings and the slower fibers carry the sensation of pain is not clarified, but apparently various thresholds for basic stimuli exist.

Crue[6] replaces the old Aristotelian concept of primary senses

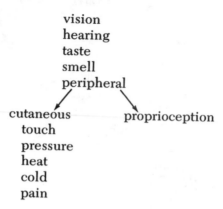

vision
hearing
taste
smell
peripheral

cutaneous — proprioception
touch
pressure
heat
cold
pain

with a classification essentially based on physical energy source:

electromagnetic
chemical
gravity
mechanical displacement
cutaneous sensibility
    mechanical
    thermal

and thus discounts nociceptive receptors. Further neurophysiologic studies reveal that T cells are capable of independent firing. This is enhanced when they are sensitized by depolarization. The T cells are postsynaptic and can be potentiated from the periphery or from central sources. In acute pain the firing of the T cells is orderly and limited, whereas in chronic pain T cell impulses can be progressive, uncontrolled, and even epileptiform.

Current concepts of pain suggest that there are neuronal pools of various levels of the central nervous system that act as pain *pattern generating mechanism*. These mechanisms become "programmed" and act as sources of pain that can be influenced by external stimuli (Fig. 135). These pools comprise a *pattern generating center* which contains the dorsal horns and all its internuncial connections. They are

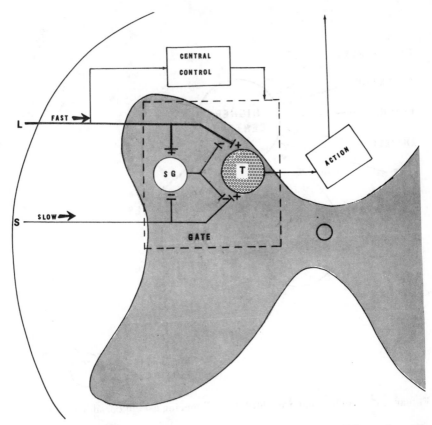

FIGURE 134. The Wahl-Melzack gate theory of pain transmission. (SG = substantia gelatinosa; T = T cells.)

influenced by peripheral impulses and also by central stimuli descending from as high as the center (Fig. 136).

These cells can be suppressed, activated, or released. These influences upon the pool can be somatic, visceral, or autonomic. There is apparently such a fine balance that a *loss* of input as well as an excess of input can result in overreaction of the pool. Loss of input can result from nerve damage with afferentation, while excess input can occur from distant tissue irritation.

In the low back pain syndromes, the peripheral irritants can result from disc herniation, foraminal root compromise, facet synovitis, myofascial irritation, or any of the numerous sites of peripheral irritation. Anxiety depression or fear can have a similar affect from descending pathways. Deafferentation from crushing or compressing a nerve by a herniated disc or any entrapment can also stimulate the pool

211

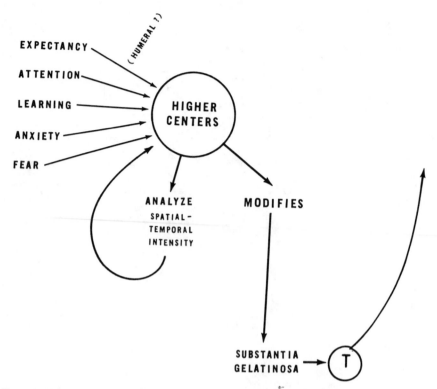

FIGURE 135. Higher center modification influencing gate in dorsal horns.

(in a "negative" way) to release the restraints upon the pool and permit chronic pain to result.

If this concept is valid there is credence in using numerous therapeutic approaches. Use of antidepressant drugs or tranquilizers may have an influence upon the *pattern generating mechanism,* used *simultaneously* with local anesthetic nerve blocks, transcutaneous nerve stimulation, sympathetic nerve blocks, and active exercises. Any and all may have a beneficial effect upon the *pool,* even though appearing to be contradictory.

The central reactivity is markedly affected by the input of the peripheral impulses. The extent of this summation is not yet validated. It is apparent that pain is not influenced exclusively by the intensity of afferent nociceptive input but is influenced markedly by higher central processes. The nociceptive afferent impulses that enter the dorsal horn of the gray matter of the cord (the "gate") in regard to tissue sites and mechanisms of causing low back pain have been discussed in previous chapters.

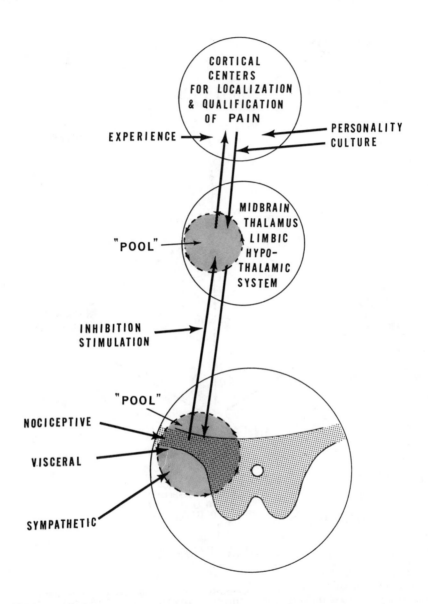

FIGURE 136. Neurone pool concept for generating pain patterns. The reverberating neurone pools that may become self-perpetuating are controlled or influenced by multiple inputs at various levels of the central nervous system. These inputs may sustain the pain behavior though no longer related to the initial nociceptive stimulus. Treatment is aimed at influencing any or all of these inputs. (Modified from Melzack, R., and Loeser, J.D.: Phantom body pain in paraplegics: evidence for a central "pattern generating mechanism" for pain. Pain 4:195-210, 1978.)

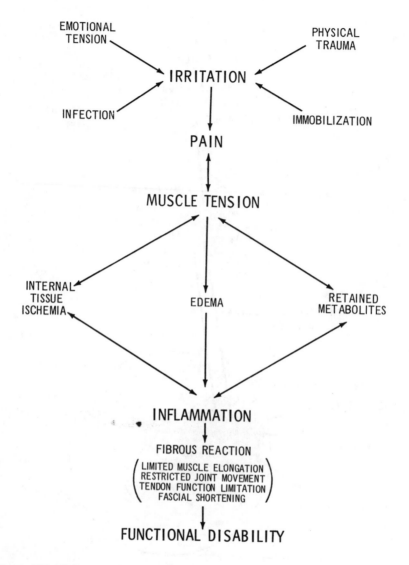

EMOTIONAL TENSION

PHYSICAL TRAUMA

INFECTION

IRRITATION

IMMOBILIZATION

PAIN

MUSCLE TENSION

INTERNAL TISSUE ISCHEMIA

EDEMA

RETAINED METABOLITES

INFLAMMATION

FIBROUS REACTION

(LIMITED MUSCLE ELONGATION
RESTRICTED JOINT MOVEMENT
TENDON FUNCTION LIMITATION
FASCIAL SHORTENING)

FUNCTIONAL DISABILITY

FIGURE 137. Schematic functional disability related to soft tissue involvement.

Pain can be mediated via the posterior primary division as well as the anterior primary division. The protective "muscle spasm" that results to prevent movement of the insulated position of the vertebral column may become the site of the nociceptive stimulus.

The ventral root, always considered principally "motor," is now known to contain many sensory fibers. Stimulation of the ventral root produces pain, muscular tension, and tenderness at the myoneural junction of that dermatome.

Sciatica, currently considered a "radiating nerve pain" from root compression at the intervertebral foramen, was originally attributed to muscle spasm. Sciatica became gradually attributable to nerve root entrapment in the intervertebral foramen when the root was found to move within the foramen on SLR. Recently this concept has been questioned when the SLR test became negative after interrupting the articular branch of the posterior primary division.[11,12] Release of muscle tension in the low back has been accepted for many years as a means of relieving backache, and consequently tension in the low back has been accepted as a cause of pain (Fig. 137).

Anxiety is often accompanied by muscular overactivity. This was postulated by Jacobson,[13] then verified in laboratory studies by Malmo[14] and by Holmes and Wolf,[15] who found that patients with backache had generalized overactivity of the trunk muscles in situations which engendered conflict, insecurity, hostility, frustration, and guilt. Patients who have been in good physical condition and well trained in their professions have been found to sustain severe low back injuries during periods of anxiety, anger, or depression.[16,17]

The psychiatric aspects of pain have gained credence in recent years and cannot be neglected in patient care. All pain has to be viewed from the patient's disease process, patient response, personality, life style and existing circumstances. Pain is a very individual matter and frequently becomes the focal point of all the patient's attention and behavior.

In *chronic pain* the "organic component" diminishes and the resultant "life style" no longer adapts properly. Recognizing this demands that treatment of chronic pain be not only to relieve or modify the organic component, but also to substitute one life style for another. The patient must be directed to a meaningful life of purpose and hope and away from pain as a "career" or life style.

The "pain-prone" patient is not always discernible during the acute painful episode. Often these patients have a history in which every episode of illness, injury, or painful experience has been a major calamity. Self-limited incidents somehow are prolonged and resistant to standard treatment procedures. Many have experienced numerous diagnostic procedures, therapeutic procedures, repeated surgical interventions, and all have failed, partially succeeded, or been followed by frequent relapse or new occurrence.

"Pain-prone patients" are often depressed, anxious, guilty, and the victims of numerous failures. Pain becomes a manner of reacting to stress, failure, or rejection. They seek medical help for support and understanding, yet too frequently are subjected to treatments for assumed organic disease, and their pain is reinforced.

215

Pain that is severe beyond what would be expected from the incidence and the physical findings, pain that persists for unexpected duration, or pain that defies acceptable treatment and doctor-patient rapport implies a significant psychiatric component.

Suspicion leading to a psychiatric diagnosis is implicated by the following:

1. Chronic anxiety. The patient is irritable, anxious, overreactive, tense, and often afflicted by painful muscular contractions of the neck, shoulders, and the *back*.
2. Misuse of medications. Chronic pain patients are often addicted to medications upon which they rely but not necessarily with relief. Medications are "needed," are numerous and various. Pain requires medication, and thus the medication rewards the pain and consequently reinforces pain.[18,19] Pain taken "as needed" fills this reinforcement role.
3. Situational stress. Pain results or has resulted from reaction to everyday stresses that are overwhelming or accumulative. The situational stress may be real or assumed.
4. Depression. The patient may subjectively manifest depression by verbalization of "blue," low, sad, "down," or depressed periods. A pessimistic view of the self or of the world may be expressed. Depression may appear as insomnia, sexual impotency, weight loss, loss of energy and thus activity, and even thoughts of suicide. The depression may be blamed on the pain rather than the pain being seen as caused by the depression.[20] Szasz[21] has used the expression "l'homme douloureaux" to describe persons who embrace a "pain career" or who play "pain games." These games are a manifestation of depression and simultaneously a challenge to the physician who attempts therapy. The patient apparently receives gratification from the physician's failure to be of help.[22] These patients also become concerned with litigation, compensation, and financial benefits that are often unrealistic in comparison to their needs or their pre-illness income.
5. Cultural factors. Studies have revealed differences of response to illness and pain in various cultures (e.g., patients of Italian and Jewish origin express pain more vividly and have a lower threshold, whereas Irish, English, and German Americans are considered more stoic and less demonstrative[23]).
6. Family influence. The relationship of family members with regard to their support or their condemnation may contribute to the severity of the patient's complaints about the alleged incapacitation. Marital relationships may often be a strong influence.

TREATMENT OF CHRONIC PAIN

Besides correcting or modifying the nociceptive components of pain, the reaction of the patient to his pain must be altered. The patients' life style must be changed to a more meaningful life pattern.

Prevention of Drug Dependency

Medications originally given "when needed" must be given at regular intervals and in decreasing strength. Thus "prn" could be changed to "q 4 hours." The patient, given the medication in an unrecognizable vehicle, must be made aware, and willing to accept, that the dosage will be gradually decreased. Drugs to "relax," then drugs to stimulate must be changed as they rarely remain effective. Antidepressants may be beneficially substituted for both or either.

Modification of Behavior

"Behavior modification" is a well-established program that rewards constructive behavior and minimizes, de-emphasizes, or ignores a pain disability reaction. "Up time" and "down time" can be recorded and the patient rewarded for increasing "up time." Rest periods have been utilized as rewards for improvement of activities.[24] Behavior modification has proven to be very effective during its initial use, but long-time benefit, in the sense of changing "coping" mechanisms, has been disappointing. Its use currently is combined with counseling to develop new coping methods.

Relaxation Techniques

The muscular tension that accompanies psychological tension *or* accompanies and intensifies organic pain can be minimized. Antianxiety drugs, such as Valium (diazepam), Librium (chlordiazepoxide), and Flexeril (cyclobenzaprine hydrochloride), have value if used during the acute phase, in controlled dosage, and with limited duration. Addiction, sedation, and depression are frequent complications arising from prolonged use.

Progressive relaxation can be taught the patient to control painful muscular tension. Hypnosis[25] has many advocates, especially in teaching self-hypnosis for relaxation. Its value on modifying severe or prolonged chronic pain is not yet well established, and practitioners skilled in its induction are not numerous.

Biofeedback of muscle potentials or EEG activities related to tension or inability to voluntarily relax painful disabling symptoms by instrumentation is gaining credence. Bodily functions considered not to be under voluntary control are now being discovered to respond to biofeedback techniques. This is particularly true of muscle tension.

Transcutaneous Electrical Nerve Stimulation

Transcutaneous electrical nerve stimulation (TENS) has been equated with use in chronic pain so that it is often withheld in acute pain where it can be very effective[26] (Fig. 138). Numerous wave forms are generated by stimulators. Several may need to be tried as patients vary in their response and benefit from TENS. The most effective wave form has not yet been established in spite of the claims of manufacturers (Fig. 139). Machines have adjustments to vary amplitude, width, type, and rate of waves. All may need to be tried before treatment is discarded or the patient is placed on a "home" machine for self-application.

TENS is not intended to cause muscular contracture, as are most electric stimulators. Because TENS is a sensory stimulator, control of intensity and wave form must be kept in mind. Most TENS machines generate wave forms of less than 100 to 150 pps and wave width of 40 to 500 pps. In applying TENS, the pulse rate is usually set at 70 to 150 pps and the amplitude gradually increased to cause the patient to experience a pleasant or tolerable sensation with no muscular contraction (Fig. 140). The amplitude of the wave is most important in depolarizing the nerve which results in nerve excitation which is what is effective in pain control. The wave pulse width is not considered pertinent. The pulse rate is also important with higher frequencies usually being more effective. This is better tolerated by the patient. Gradual adjustment of the amplitude and frequency should be attempted by the therapist, *not by the patient.*

The patient must be informed of what TENS is and what it may do for the pain:

1. give complete relief of varying duration;
2. give only partial or temporary relief;
3. be of no value.

Before accepting failure, the proper wave amplitude, frequency (rate), and pulse width must be established with numerous trials. The proper site of application must be determined, and different instruments may need to be tried.

The site of application of TENS on the body surface is not standardized and may require some searching. The precise site may prove to be at the site of pain which may be at a motor point of a muscle, may

218

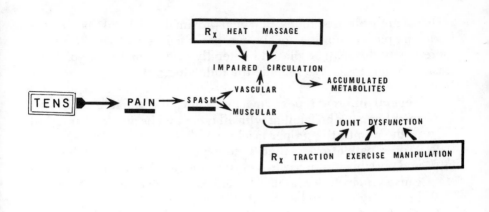

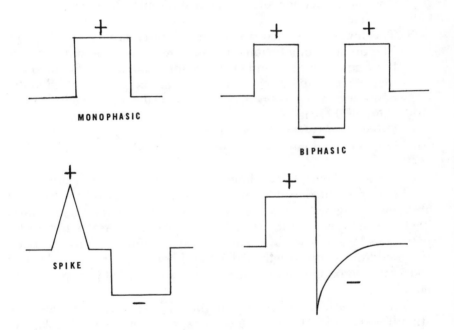

FIGURE 139. Wave forms of TENS.

be over branches of the peripheral nerve innervating the painful site, or may be at the emergence of a nerve root in the paraspinous region.[27] The clinical examination gives an indication of whether pain is local or referred, but often both may need to be considered in the application of TENS (Fig. 141).

Use of multiple electrodes, in which proximal and distal (local) electrodes are placed simultaneously, may prove to be effective. The two or more electrodes may be placed bilaterally or proximally and distally. Basic guidelines for use include the following:[28-31]

1. Several different types of machines must be available, and a staff member must be familiar with all types and be able to employ all of them until the proper machine is found.
2. Proper patient orientation as to expected use, possible benefit, and possible minor hazards must be given. The electrode gel may cause skin irritation, as may the adhesive or plastic tape: either, or both, may need to be changed.
3. The beneficial current must be discovered by trial and error as to wave amplitude, width, and frequency.
4. The most effective site of application must be discovered and then charted.
5. The duration of each treatment must be ascertained and recorded. The duration of a treatment benefit must be determined before the frequency of treatment is decided upon. It is important to instruct the patient who may ultimately be given a machine for home use. These facts also have clinical significance as to the value of this modality.
6. Other forms of treatment such as exercise, proper activity instruction, and medication can also be used simultaneously.

Loss or lack of peripheral stimuli may permit the "pattern generating mechanism" of the dorsal horn of the gray matter to persist in (central) abnormal firing patterns. Deafferentiation of peripheral impulses has been shown to produce abnormal bursts of firing in dorsal horn cells for periods as long as 180 days. This central abnormal activity has been recorded from lamina 5 cells in the dorsal horn: a neuronal pool that is considered to be involved in sensory transmission of pain-producing impulses.[32]

Pain can be intercepted or modified by decreasing nociceptive stimuli with anesthetic nerve block or sympathetic nerve blocks, but when there is deafferentiation with resultant anesthesia or hypesthesia, pain may be intensified. This has been examplified in phantom pain, in paraplegia, and in patients with complete nerve interruption.[33]

Partially interrupted peripheral nerves have been known to result in severe causalgic pain. This can be considered as a result of the dorsal horn "pattern generating mechanism" receiving confusing messages.

Combining anesthetic nerve blocks and sympathetic nerve blocks with electrical nerve stimulation appears to be paradoxical except when viewed from the concept.

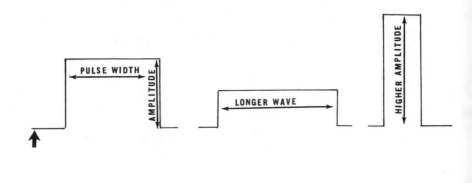

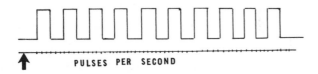

FIGURE 140. Characteristics of TENS application.

PSYCHIATRIC TREATMENT AND COUNSELING

It is evident that there is a difference between organic pain and "suffering." The complaint of the patient frequently may not correlate with the degree of impairment or with the extent of improvement from any program. Pain can be equated to the nociceptive insult, but suffering is not necessarily so equated. Suffering is influenced by learned behavior and usually has secondary gains: psychological needs, security, dependency, and possibly financial awards. These latter factors must be considered along with treatment of organic causative factors.

In the game of "painsmanship" the patient's aim is to produce undiagnosable pain and unrelievable suffering: this creates meaning for his life and power to control his environment. Chronic pain may constitute a "career."

MALINGERING

The use of the term *malingering* cannot be avoided in a discussion of low back pain with or without subjective sciatica. If malingering is alleged, the statement implies that symptoms have been intentionally

221

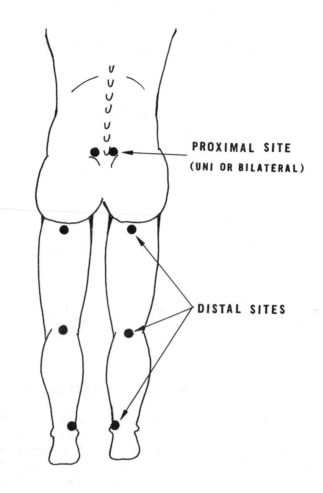

FIGURE 141. Sites of usual application of TENS.

falsified for fraudulent gains and that the symptoms have no organic or psychological neurophysiologic basis. This places the diagnosis of malingering more within the realm of accusation.

True malingering is considered to be rare and, by some, to be nonexistent. Differentiation is difficult to achieve in relation to anxiety and conversion hysteria. No laboratory or psychological battery of tests can clearly delineate a suspected malingerer. The secondary gain expected, or desired, by the chronically painful patient and the mode of life accepted by the patient must be discovered, explored, and every attempt made to modify that unacceptable activity.[34]

CONCLUSION

Treating a patient complaining of chronic low back pain requires a thorough evaluation of (1) the person suffering; (2) the secondary gains from this disability, whether financial or personal; (3) the personality of the sufferer; and (4) the physical examination to determine nociceptive sites.

All aspects need to be involved in a treatment program. These include:

1. Eradication or minimizing any "organic" component of tissue irritation by
   a. nerve blocks;
   b. exercises;
   c. medication;
   d. bracing;
   e. sympathetic nerve blocks;
   f. modalities such as heat, ice, massage, TENS, etc.;
   g. surgery.
2. Progressive relaxation.
3. Hypnosis.
4. Behavior modification.
5. Counseling.
6. Vocational counseling.

The long-term aim with patients suffering from chronic disability low back pain is primarily to provide them with skills and techniques to cope more adequately with their pain problems. As total relief of chronic pain often may be unattainable, the goal can only be for patients to live as full and as normal a life as is possible "in spite of their pain."

REFERENCES

1. Cailliet, R.: Soft Tissue Pain and Disability. F.A. Davis, Philadelphia, 1977.
2. Brena, S.F.: Chronic Pain: America's Hidden Epidemic. Atheneum/SMI, New York, 1978.
3. Shanfeld, S.B., and Killingsworth, R.N.: The psychiatric aspects of pain. Psychiat. Ann. 7(1):24-35, 1977.
4. Steinbach, R.A., et al.: Chronic low back pain: "low-back loser." Postgrad. Med. 53:135-138, 1973.

5. Bonica, J.J.: The Management of Pain. Lea & Febiger, Philadelphia, 1953.
6. Crue, B.L.: Pain. Bull. Los Angeles Co. Med. Assoc., Oct. 4, 1973, pp. 10-15.
7. Forst, J.J.: Contribution a l'etude clinique de la sciatique. Paris Thése, No. 33, 1881.
8. Laségue, C.: Considerations sur la sciatique. Arch. Gen. Med. 2 (Serie 6, Tome 4): 558-580, 1864.
9. Minter, W.J., and Barr, J.S.: Rupture of the intervertebral disk with involvement of the spinal canal. N. Engl. J. Med. 211-210, 215, 1934.
10. King, J.S., and Lagger, R.: Sciatica viewed as a referred pain syndrome. Surg. Neurol. 5:46-50, 1976.
11. Rees, W.S.: Multiple bilateral subcutaneous rhizolysis of segmental nerves in the treatment of the intervertebral disc syndrome. Ann. Gen. Pract. 26:126-127, 1971.
12. Shealy, C.N.: Facets in back and sciatic pain: a new approach to a major pain syndrome. Minn. Med. 57:199-203, 1974.
13. Jacobson, E.: Electrical measurements of neuromuscular states during mental activities. I. Imagination of movement involving skeletal muscles. Am. J. Physiol. 91:567-608, 1930.
14. Malmo, R.B., and Shagass, C.: Physiologic studies of reaction to stress in anxiety and early schizophrenia. Psychosomat. Med. 11:9, 25, 1949.
15. Holmes, T.H., and Wolff, H.G.: Life situations, emotions and backache. Psychosomat. Med. 14:18, 1952.
16. Hirschfeld, A.H., and Behan, R.C.: The accident process. J.A.M.A. 186:193-199, 1963.
17. Holmes, T., and Rahe, R.: The social readjustment rating scale. J. Psychosom. Res. 11:213-218, 1967.
18. Fordyce, W.E., et al.: Operant conditioning method for managing chronic pain. Postgrad. Med. 53:123-128, 1973.
19. Fordyce, W.E., et al.: Operant conditioning in the treatment of chronic pain. Arch. Phys. Med. Rehab. 54:399-408, 1973.
20. Steinbach, R.A.: Pain and depression, in Kiev, A. (ed.): Somatic Manifestations of Depressive Disorders. Excerpta Medica, Elsevier, New York, 1974.
21. Szasz, T.: The psychology of persistent pain: a portrait of l'homme douloureux, in Soulairac, A., et al. (eds.): Pain. Academic Press, New York, 1968.
22. Steinbach, R.A., and Rush, T.N.: Alternatives to the pain career. Psychotherapy: Theory, Research and Practice 10 (1973), 321-324.
23. Zborowski, M.: People in Pain. Jossey-Bass, San Francisco, 1967.
24. Fordyce, W.E.: Behavioral Methods for Chronic Pain and Illness. C.V. Mosby, St. Louis, 1976.
25. Finer, B.: Clinical use of hypnosis in pain management, in Bonica, J.J. (ed.): Pain. (Advances in Neurology, Vol. 4) Raven Press, New York, 1974.
26. Lampe, G.N.: Introduction to the use of transcutaneous electrical nerve stimulation device. Phys. Therap. 58 (12):1450-1466, 1978.
27. Mannheimer, J.S.: Electrode placements for transcutaneous electrical nerve stimulation. Phys. Therap. 58 (12):1455-1462, 1978.
28. Steinbach, R.: Pain patients: traits and treatment. Academic Press, New York, 1974.
29. Szasz, T.S.: The painful person. Lancet, January 1968, p. 18.
30. Newman, R.I., Seres, J.L., Yospe, L.P., and Garlington, B.: Multidisciplinary treatment of chronic pain: long-term follow-up of low back pain patients. Pain 4:283-292, 1978.
31. Melzack, R., and Loeser, J.D.: Phantom body pain in paraplegics: evidence for a central "pattern generating mechanism" for pain. Pain 4:195-210, 1978.
32. Hillman, P., and Wall, P.D.: Inhibitory and excitatory factors influencing the receptive fields of lamina 5 spinal cord cells. Exp. Brain Res. 9:284-306, 1969.
33. Davis, L., and Martin, J.: Studies upon spinal cord injuries. II. The nature and treatment of pain. J. Neurosurg. 4:483-491, 1947.
34. Shaw, R.S.: Pathological malingering: the painful disabled extremity. N. Engl. J. Med. 271:22-26, 1964.

BIBLIOGRAPHY

Kirgis, H.D.: Problems in the management of the "compensation" patient with lumbar disk syndrome. Southern Med. J. 57(10):1152-1156, 1964.

Melzack, R.: The Puzzle of Pain. Basic Books, New York, 1973.

Melzack, R., and Perry, C.: Self-regulation of pain: the use of alpha-feedback and hypnotic training for the control of chronic pain. Exp. Neurol. 46:452-469, 1975.

Nathan, P.W.: The gate control theory of pain: a critical review. Brain 99:123-158, 1976.

Papper, S.: The undesirable patient (editorial). J. Chron. Dis. 22:777-779, 1970.

Shaw, R.S.: Pathological malingering. N. Engl. J. Med. 271:22-26, 1964.

Wolkind, S.N., and Forrest, A.J.: Low back pain: a psychiatric investigation. Postgrad. Med. J. 48:76-79, 1972.

Index